Adjunctive medical therapy of acromegalic patients

CLINICAL RESEARCH SERIES

The aim of this series is to draw attention to results of clinical research projects of interest to physicians in the field of internal medicine and related disciplines.
The editors hope that by reaching a wide audience, it will increase and facilitate practical application of recent findings.

Adjunctive medical therapy of acromegalic patients

J.W.R. Nortier

1984
FORIS PUBLICATIONS
Dordrecht-Holland/Cinnaminson-U.S.A.

Published by:
Foris Publications Holland
P.O. Box 509
3300 AM Dordrecht, The Netherlands

Sole distributor for the U.S.A. and Canada:
Foris Publications U.S.A.
Cinnaminson N.J. 08077
U.S.A.

ISBN 90 6765 093 5

Printed in the Netherlands by ICG Printing, Dordrecht.

Aan Josien,
Lodewijk en Susan

List of abbreviations

ACTH	: adrenocorticotroph hormone
CRF	: corticotroph releasing factor
E_1	: oestrone
E_2	: oestradiol
FSH	: follicular stimulating hormone
GH	: growth hormone
GRF	: growth hormone releasing factor
h	: hour
IGF-I	: insulin-like growth factor-I
IGF-II	: insulin-like growth factor-II
IRP	: international reference preparation
Irr	: external irradiation
LH	: luteinizing hormone
LHRH	: luteinizing hormone releasing hormone
MRC	: Medical Research Council
MW	: molecular weight
n.s.	: not significant
OGTT	: oral glucose tolerance test
Prl	: prolactin
SD	: standard deviation
SEM	: standard error of the mean
Sm-A	: somatomedin-A
Sm-C	: somatomedin-C
T_4	: thyroxin
TFS	: transfrontal surgery
TRH	: thyrotrophin releasing hormone
TSH	: thyrotrophin stimulating hormone
TSS	: transsphenoidal surgery
Vo	: void volume
Ve	: elution volume
Vt	: total volume
VIP	: vasoactive intestinal polypeptide

Contents

CHAPTER I

Introduction

The clinical and biochemical studies described in this thesis were performed to evaluate the medical therapy of acromegaly. After a short outline of the historical background, epidemiology and pathogenesis of the disorder, the various therapeutic modalities are discussed. Finally the questions which we tried to answer will be defined.

HISTORICAL BACKGROUND

Acromegaly was the first pituitary disorder to be clinically recognized by Pierre Marie in 1886 (1). In this earliest paper on the subject, Marie did not find any pathological cause of the abnormalities he observed. He named the condition after the Greek "akron" (= extremity) and "megas" (= great). The role of the pituitary gland was suspected on the basis of necropsy studies and in 1900 Benda (2) advanced the idea that acromegaly was the result of hyperfunction of cells containing eosinophylic granules. Cushing (3) reinforced this belief in 1909 based on clinical and pathological studies and on the observation of remission in symptoms of some cases after partial removal of the pars anterior. Evans (4) in 1921 gave experimental support to this hypothesis by demonstrating that parenteral injection of an extract of the anterior pituitary can produce gigantism in rats. Li (5) first reported the isolation of growth hormone (GH) in a highly purified form from bovine pituitary glands in 1944. In 1956 human GH was isolated in a pure form and was shown to be structurally different from bovine GH (6). The final revision of its structure was published in 1971 (7). It is a single chain polypeptide with a molecular weight of 21.500 containing 191 amino-acids residues with two disulfide bridges. The development of a radioimmunoassay for GH by Hunter and Greenwood (8) in 1962 has contributed to confirm or refute a clinical diagnosis of acromegaly, to assess the response to treatment and to increase the understanding of its etiology.

EPIDEMIOLOGY

Pituitary adenomas are common, being found in 15-25% of autopsies (9-11) but GH secreting adenomas probably account for a small part of these. Tumours causing acromegaly are usually diagnosed clinically as their manifestations are so apparent during life. Unlike prolactin-secreting tumours and so-called non-functioning tumours, GH secreting adenomas are rarely discovered routinely at autopsy. In a community survey Alexander et al. (12) studied a population of 3.1 million in the Newcastle region during a period of 11 years and concluded that a firm diagnosis of acromegaly had been made in 164 patients. Based on these data, the annual incidence of acromegaly is approximately 3 per million and the prevalence of diagnosed cases may be as high as 40 per million. In view of the relative stability of the population studied, these figures are probably representative for the true incidence of the disorder in the population and can also be applied to the Netherlands.

PATHOPHYSIOLOGY

On clinical and pathological evidence it cannot be decided whether GH-secreting pituitary tumours are caused by a primary pituitary defect, by defective hypothalamic control or by a combination of both factors.

The following lines of evidence suggest that acromegaly is a primary pituitary disease:

a. Histology of pituitary tissue surrounding the focal GH-secreting adenoma is normal (13,14). This favours the concept of the tumour arising from a locally transformed cell within the pituitary without stimulation of excessive hypothalamic growth hormone releasing factor (GRF).
b. The discovery and characterization of mixed GH and Prl cell tumours associated with acromegaly. The neoplastic transformation and proliferation of Prl secreting cells is unlikely to be caused by excessive secretion of hypothalamic GRF.
c. Following selective removal of GH secreting tumours, in some cases basal GH levels have returned to normal levels (15-21), qualitative GH responses to provocative stimuli have been reported to revert to normal (22) and also normal 24 hour GH secretion patterns with nocturnal GH rises during deep sleep have been observed (23).

On the other hand, there is also evidence that acromegaly may result from a defect in the inhibitory and stimulatory hypothalamic control of GH secretion, respectively by somatostatin (24,25) and by GRF (26-30):

a. GH containing pituitary adenomas have been described in association with hypothalamic tumours presumably secreting GRF (31-33).
b. Serum obtained from patients with acromegaly exhibited GRF activity in an **in vitro** bio-assay (34-36).

c. After surgical removal of GH secreting adenomas even though basal GH levels return to normal, qualitative GH responses to provocative stimuli frequently remain abnormal suggesting an intrinsic hypothalamic disorder not corrected by surgical removal of the adenoma (37).
d. Some acromegalic patients exhibit normal GH responses to pharmacological stimuli (α-adrenergic blockade, β-adrenergic stimulation) and physiological stimuli (stress, sleep) suggesting that GH secretion is not autonomous and is apparently regulated by physiological mechanisms (38,39). This is in contrast to the abnormal GH suppression by L-Dopa (40,41) and the hypersecretion of GH after TRH (42,43).
e. Recently, a patient has been described with acromegaly due to somatotroph hyperplasia, caused by ectopic GRF production from a pancreatic tumour. Paradoxical stimulation of GH by glucose and TRH and suppression by dopamine reverted to normal after the source of ectopic GRF production had been removed (44). This suggests that the abnormal GH response may be due to altered pituitary regulation by excessive GRF or decreased somatostatin or both. Alternatively, the high levels of circulating GH could have been responsible for the observed paradoxical responses.
f. Primary cultures of rat (45) and human (46) somatotroph adenoma cells have recently been shown to respond to GRF suggesting the presence of GRF receptors on human GH adenoma cells.
g. The dynamics of **in vitro** GH secretion by GH adenoma tissue are similar to those observed in culture of normal adult and fetal tissues (47). Thus, abnormalities of secretory dynamics in acromegaly are probably not due to alterations at the pituitary level but due to central defects in GH regulation.

In summary, there is evidence that in some GH cell adenomas a certain degree of central hypothalamic control is maintained, while in others this control is distorted.

In view of the conflicting data a final conclusion with respect to the pathogenesis of acromegaly is not justified.

DIAGNOSIS

The main clinical features are listed in Table 1. Diagnosis is made by the typical changes in body configuration, [. . .] demonstration of a pituitary tumor by X-ray or visual field defects, and most importantly by an elevated basal plasma GH level which does not decrease during a standard glucose tolerance test, although in some acromegalic patients a decrease has been seen. In addition a paradoxical rise of the plasma GH level after administration of TRH or LHRH can be found in some patients.

Because the skeletal changes are permanent, it is important in the treated as well as the untreated case to determine whether there is continual hypersecretion of GH, or whether a deficiency of GH and perhaps of other hormones has resulted from pituitary destruction from pressure, hemorrhage or earlier therapy. Activity of the process is implied by continued skeletal and soft-tissue growth, by the presence of diabetes mellitus or impaired glucose tolerance, by elevated levels of serum inorganic phosphorus and alkaline phosphatase, and by increased excretion of hydroxyproline in the urine.

Table 1. Main clinical features (derived from 5 major studies 1962–1981)

Acral enlargement and soft tissue overgrowth	100%
Hyperhidrosis	65–88%
Headache	50–73%
Paraesthesiae	49–79%
Diabetes mellitus and impaired glucose tolerance	27–60%
Cardiovascular problems	12–34%
Hypertension	18–32%
Goitre	18–32%
Menstrual disorders	32–80%
Decreased libido and impotence	27–46%
Visual field defects	6–25%

TREATMENT

In acromegaly a reduced life expectancy has been reported due to cardiovascular, cerebrovascular and respiratory disease (12,48). Mortality rates are higher for untreated than for treated patients. Therefore, there is a consensus that once acromegaly is diagnosed, treatment must be instituted which is aimed at normalization of the GH secretion, the reduction of tumour mass and the preservation of normal pituitary function. As the spontaneous course of the disease is not accurately known, this factor has also to be taken into account when the effects of various forms of treatment are assessed.

SURGERY

Transsphenoidal surgery with the aim of selective adenomectomy is the most effective form of treatment (49). However, the cure rate assessed by dynamic studies of post-operative GH secretion is still low as acromegalics have usually progressed beyond the micro-adenoma stage by the time the condition is diagnosed and as the sellar dura or parasellar structures are frequently infiltrated by adenomatous tissue (15,23,50,51).

RADIOTHERAPY

External irradiation has a place in the therapeutic management of acromegaly for patients who are not cured by surgery. In addition, it can be considered as a primary form of treatment in older patients with mild clinical and biochemical activity and in patients who are poor surgical risks. This treatment may take up to 10 years to be optimally effective in suppressing GH secretion (52-54).

Interstitial pituitary irradiation with Yttrium (90Y) or irradiation with a beam of heavy alpha particles is only available in a few centres (55,56). The maximal effect on suppression of GH secretion occurs within 2 years after its administration. But with these forms of therapy a high incidence of hypopituitarism has been reported (55,57).

MEDICAL THERAPY

The possibility of additional medical therapy has received much attention when it was discovered in 1972 that L-dopa (40) and in 1974 that the dopamine agonist bromocriptine (58) decreased GH levels in a number of acromegalic patients. This stands in marked contrast to their stimulatory effect on GH secretion in normal subjects (59,60), due to a stimulation of dopamine receptors in the central nervous system. The reduction of GH secretion in acromegaly is probably mediated by dopamine dependent mechanisms at the pituitary level. This paradoxical effect of dopamine as well as other aberrant responses to TRH (42), LHRH (61), VIP (62) or CRF (63) may also be caused by lack of receptor specificity of some pituitary cells.

By far the greatest clinical experience in the medical treatment of acromegaly has been obtained with the dopamine agonist bromocriptine (64-74). Good results have been reported by a number of investigators by evaluating the GH suppressive effect of bromocriptine with GH measurements at fixed intervals during the day (64,65,68-72,74). Negative results have been reported in a recent double-blind cross-over study (73) and in two earlier studies (66,67). In these studies the GH suppressive effect was evaluated by measuring plasma GH levels either during oral glucose tolerance tests (OGTT's) or only during 6 hours of the day. The use of an OGTT has been criticized as the physiological control of GH is not tested by this method (75). Moreover, as bromocriptine has a short duration of action, the time interval between the last dose of bromocriptine and the performance of an OGTT may be critical. The criteria used to define the clinical and plasma GH response to chronic bromocriptine therapy are not uniform. In most studies a decrease of the mean plasma GH level during the day of at least 50% is considered as a partial response and these patients are then called "responders". Complete responses with plasma GH levels during the day below 5 mU/l occur in a minority of patients (less than 15%). It seems therefore appropriate to define a 50% decrease of the mean plasma GH level during the day as a positive response. In this way the "response rate" to chronic bromocriptine therapy varies from 50-90%.

Improvement of subjective clinical symptoms and of objective criteria of clinical activity such as urinary hydroxyproline excretion, glucose tolerance and ring size has been noted out of proportion to the fall in GH in several studies (70,74,76,79). Explanations offered for these discrepancies between the clinical and GH response to chronic bromocriptine therapy have been a selective reduction of the somatomedins, particularly somatomedin-C, through which GH exerts its growth promoting effects and a preferential reduction of the biologically more active monomeric form of GH.

A good correlation has been found between the plasma GH response to a single dose of bromocriptine and to chronic bromocriptine therapy (68,71,79). Responsiveness to bromocriptine in the acute test is often accompanied by a paradoxical rise of GH after administration of TRH (58,71). The responsiveness to TRH and acute bromocriptine tests has been related to hyperprolactinaemia or to the ability of the adenoma cells to synthesize Prl (80,81) although this is not generally accepted (82,83). Also, a similarity in the GH lowering effect of dopamine and somatostatin has been reported (84,85). The degree of GH suppression during somatostatin infusion may also have predictive value with respect to the results of chronic bromocriptine therapy. No investigations are reported in which all these tests have been compared in order to find the combination with the highest predictive value.

It is thought that in patients in whom dopamine agonists fail, hypothalamic control of GH secretion could still be present and that the GH levels could then be reduced by anti-dopaminergic agents such as pimozide (86).

Based on the fore-going the following questions were defined:

1. Is the result different if the GH suppressive effect of bromocriptine is evaluated by measurement of plasma GH levels at fixed intervals during the day or if plasma GH is measured during OGTT's and how critical is the time-interval between the last dose of bromocriptine and the performance of an OGTT? (Chapter II).
2. What is the effect of chronic bromocriptine therapy on the GH secretion and on subjective and objective criteria of clinical activity in patients with still active acromegaly after previous pituitary surgery and/or radiotherapy? (Chapter III).
3. What is the value of four predictive criteria either in combination or separately (i.e. acute bromocriptine test, TRH-test, somatostatin infusion and basal Prl) with respect to the effect of chronic bromocriptine therapy on the GH secretion? (Chapter III).
4. Is measurement of somatomedin-C superior to measurement of plasma GH levels during the day in the assessment of the clinical response to

chronic bromocriptine therapy in acromegaly? (Chapter IV).

5. What is the influence of chronic bromocriptine therapy in acromegaly on the different molecular forms of GH? Does the change of the biologically most active monomeric form of GH provide a better correlation than the change of total GH to the clinical response and to the change of somatomedin-C? (Chapter V).
6. Is there a fundamental difference in the degree of hypothalamic dopaminergic control of GH – or Prl secretion between bromocriptine sensitive and bromocriptine insensitive acromegalic patients? (Chapter VI).
7. Does acromegaly always show clinical, biochemical and radiological progression when treatment is withheld? (Chapter VII).

REFERENCES

1. Marie P (1886). Sur deux cas d'acromégalie: hypertrophie singulière non congenitale des extrémities superieures, inférieures et céphalique. Rev Med (Paris) 6: 297-333.
2. Benda C (1900). Beiträge zur normalen und pathologischen Histologie der menschlichen Hypophysis cerebri. Berl klin Wchnschr 36: 1205-1210.
3. Cushing H (1909). The hypophysis cerebri: clinical aspects of hyperpituitarism and hypopituitarism. JAMA 53: 249-255.
4. Evans HM, Long JA (1921). The effect of the anterior lobe administered intraperitoneally upon growth, maturity and oestrous cycle of the rat. Anat Rec 21: 62-63.
5. Li CH & Evans HM (1944). Isolation of pituitary growth hormone. Science 99: 183-184.
6. Li CH & Papkoff (1956). Preparation and properties of growth hormone from human and monkey pituitary glands. Science 124: 1293-1294.
7. Li CH & Dixon JS (1971). Human pituitary growth hormone XXXII. The primary structure of the hormone: revision. Arch Biochem Biophys 146: 233-236.
8. Hunter WM & Greenwood FC (1962). Preparation of iodine-131 labelled human growth hormone of high specific activity. Nature 194: 495-496.
9. Costello RJ (1936). Subclinical adenoma of the pituitary gland. Am J Pathol 12: 205-215.
10. Burrow GN, Wortzman G, Rewcastle NB, Holgate RC, Kovacs K (1981). Microadenomas of the pituitary and abnormal sellar tomograms in an unselected autopsy series. N Engl J med 304: 156-158.
11. Gold EB (1981). Epidemiology of pituitary adenomas. Epidemiol Rev 3: 163-183.
12. Alexander L, Appleton D, Hall R, Ross WM, Wilkinson R (1980). Epidemiology of acromegaly in the Newcastle region. Clin Endocrinol (Oxf) 12: 71-79.
13. Saeger W (1977). Die Morphologie der pareadenomatosen Adenohypophyse. Ein Beitrag zur Pathogenese der Hypophysenadenome. Virchows Arch Pathol Anat 372: 299-314.
14. Landolt AM (1979). Pituitary adenomas. Clinicomorphologic correlations. J Histochem Cytochem 27: 1395-1397.
15. Arafah BUM, Bradkey JS, Kaufman B, Velasco M, Manni A, Pearson OH (1980). Transsphenoidal microsurgery in the treatment of acromegaly and gigantism. J Clin Endocrinol Metab 50: 578-585.
16. Allen JP, Cook DM, Greer MA (1973). Evidence that acromegaly is not a hypothalamic disease. Trans Assoc Am Physicians 80: 272-283.
17. Hoyte KM, Martin JB (1975). Recovery from paradoxical growth hormone responses in acromegaly after transsphenoidal selective adenomectomy. J Clin Endocrinol Metab 41: 656-659.

18. Kinnman J (1976). The prognosis in acromegaly treated by transanthro-sphenoidal operation. Acta Otolaryngol 82: 420-430.
19. Hardy J (1979). Transsphenoidal microsurgical treatment of pituitary tumors. In: Linfoot JA (ed). Recent Advances in the Diagnosis and Treatment of Pituitary Tumors. Raven Press, New York, pp 375-388.
20. Wanski ZJ, Robinson AG, Jannetta PJ (1979). Selective total removal of a growth hormone-secreting adenoma: evidence that acromegaly is a primary pituitary disease. Metabolism 28: 624-628.
21. Baskin DS, Boggan JE, Wilson CB (1982). Transsphenoidal microsurgical removal of growth hormone-secreting pituitary adenomas. J Neurosurg 56: 634-641.
22. Faglia G, Parachi A, Ferrari C, Beck-Peccoz P (1978). Evaluation of the results of transsphenoidal surgery in acromegaly by assessment of the growth hormone response to thyrotropin-releasing hormone. Clin Endocrinol (Oxf) 8: 373-380.
23. Jaquet P, Guibout M, Jaquet C, Grisoli F, Devolx BC, Dumas D, Bert J (1980). Circadian regulation of growth hormone secretion after treatment in acromegaly. J Clin Endocrinol Metab 50: 322-328.
24. Brazeau P, Vale W, Burgus R, Ling N, Butcher M, Rivier J, Guillemin R (1973). Hypothalamic polypeptide that inhibits the secretion of immunoreactive pituitary growth hormone. Science 179: 77-79.
25. Krulich L, Dharlwal APS, McCann SM (1968). Stimulatory and inhibitory effects of purified hypothalamic extracts on growth hormone release from rat pituitary in vitro. Endocrinology 83: 783-790.
26. Thorner MO, Spiess J, Vance ML, Rogol AD, Kaiser KL, Webster JD, Rivier J, Borges JL, Bloom SR, Cronin MJ, Evans WS, Macleod RM, Vale W (1983). Human pancreatic growth-hormone-releasing factor selectively stimulates growth hormone secretion in man. Lancet i: 24-28.
27. Daughaday WH, Cryer PE, Jacobs LS (1973). The role of the hypothalamus in the pathogenesis of pituitary tumors. In: Kohler PO, Ross GT (eds). Diagnosis and Treatment of Pituitary Tumors. Excerpta Medica, Amsterdam, pp 26-34.
28. Martin JB (1973), Neural regulation of growth hormone secretion. N Engl J Med 288: 1384-1393.
29. Martin JB (1980). Functions of central nervous system neurotransmitters in regulation of growth hormone secretion. Fed Proc 39: 2902-2907.
30. Reichlin S (1980). Anatomical and physiological basis of the hypothalamus-pituitary regulation. In: Post KD, Jackson IMD, Rechlin S (eds). The Pituitary Adenoma. Plenum Pres, New York, pp 3-27.
31. Müller W 1959. Uber das gemeinsame Vorkommen eines Hypophysenadenoms mit einem Gangliocytom in zwei Fallen. Ein Beitrag zur Frage der Neurosekretion. Acta Neurochirurg 7: 13-29.
32. Asa SL, Bilbao JM, Kovacs K, Linfoot JA (1980). Hypothalamic neuronal hamartoma associated with pituitary growth hormone cell adenoma and acromegaly. Acta Neuropathol (Berl) 52: 231-234.
33. Rhodes RH, Dusseau JJ, Boyd AS Jr, Knigge KM (1982). Intrasellar neural-adenohypophyseal choristoma. A morphological and immunocytochemical study. J Neuropathol Exp Neurol 41: 267-280.
34. Stachura ME, Frohman LA, Dhariwal APS (1971). Effect of purified hypothalamic extract acromegalic plasma on growth hormone synthesis and secretion in vitro. Endocrinology 88: A-81.
35. Hagen TC, Lawrence AM, Kirsteins L (1971). In vitro release of monkey pituitary growth hormone by acromegalic plasma. J Clin Endocrinol 33: 448-451.
36. Hagen TC, Lawrence AM, Kacherian EL, Kirsteins L (1972). A dialyzable heat stable factor in acromegalic plasma associated with increased in vitro growth hormone release. Proc Soc Exp Biol Med 141: 536-539.

37. Frohman LA (1981). Disease of the anterior pituitary. In: Felig P, Baxter J, Broadus AE, Frohman LA (eds). Endocrinology and Metabolism. McGraw-Hill, New York, p 204.
38. Lawrence AM, Goldfine ID, Korstein L (1970). Growth hormone dynamics in acromegaly. J Clin Endocrinol Metab 31: 239-247.
39. Cryer PE, Daughaday WH (1974). Adrenergic modulation of growth hormone secretion in acromegaly: suppression during phentolamine and phentoxamine-isoproterenol administration. J Clin Endocrinol Metab 39: 658-663.
40. Liuzzi A, Chiodini PG, Botalla L, Cremascoli G, Silvestrini F (1972). Inhibitory effects of L-dopa on GH release in acromegalic patients. J Clin Endocrinol Metab 35: 941-943.
41. Martin JB (1979) Pathophysiology of growth hormone regulation. In: Tolis G, Labrie F, Martin JB, Naftolin F (eds). Clinical Neuroendocrinology, a pathophysiological approach. Raven Press, New York, p 437.
42. Irie M, Tsushima T (1972). Increase in serum growth hormone concentration following thyrotropin releasing hormone injection in patients with acromegaly or gigantism. J Clin Endocrinol Metab 35: 97-100.
43. Gomez-Pan A, Tunbridge WMG, Duns A (1975). Hypothalamic hormone interaction in acromegaly. Clin Endocrinol (Oxf) 4: 455-460.
44. Thorner MO, Perryman RL, Cronin MJ, Rogol AD, Draznin M, Johanson A, Vale W, Horvath E, Kovacs K (1982). Somatotroph hyperplasia. Successful treatment of acromegaly by removal of a pancreatic islet tumor secreting a growth hormone-releasing factor. J Clin Invest 70: 965-977.
45. Cronin MJ, Rogol AD, Dabney LG, Thorner MO (1982). Selective growth hormone and cyclic AMP stimulating activity is present in a human pancreatic islet cell tumor. J Clin Endocrinol Metab 55: 381-383.
46. Webb CB, Thominet JL, Frohman LA (1983). Ectopic growth hormone releasing factor stimulates growth hormone release from human somatotroph adenomas in vitro. J Clin Endocrinol Metab 56: 417-419.
47. Marcovitz S, Goodyer G, Guyda H, Gardiner RJ, Hardy J (1982). Comparative study of human fetal, normal adult and somatotrophic adenoma pituitary function in tissue culture. J Clin Endocrinol Metab 54: 6-16.
48. Wright AD. Hill DM, Lowy C, Russell Fraser T (1970). Mortality in acromegaly. Q J Med 34: 1-16.
49. Quabbe HJ (1982). Treatment of acromegaly by transsphenoidal operation, 90-Yttrium implantation and bromocriptine: results in 230 patients. Clin Endocrinol (Oxf) 16: 107-119.
50. Laws ER, Piepgras DG, Randall RV, Abboud CF (1979). Neurosurgical management of acromegaly. J Neurosurg 50: 454-461.
51. Hulting AL, Werner S, Wersäll J (1982). Normal growth hormone secretion is rare after microsurgical normalization of growth hormone levels in acromegaly. Acta Med Scand 212: 401-405.
52. Eastman RC, Gordon P, Roth J (1979). Conventional supervoltage irradiation is an effective treatment for acromegaly. J Clin Endocrinol Metab 48: 931-940.
53. Lawrence AM, Pinsky SM, Goldfine MD (1971). Conventional radiation therapy in acromegaly. Arch Intern Med 128: 369-371.
54. Feek CM, Mc Lelland J, Seth J, Toft AD, Irvine WJ, Padfield PL, Edwards RW (1984). How effective is external pituitary irradiation for growth hormone-secreting tumors? Clin Endocrinol (Oxf) 20: 401-408.
55. Cassar J, Doyle FH, Banks LM, Jadresic A, Mashiter K, Joplin GF (1981), Interstitial pituitary irradiation with 90 Y for the treatment of acromegaly. A reappraisal. Acta Endocrinol (Copenh) 96: 295-300.
56. Lawrence JH, Tobias CA, Linfoot JA, Borns JL, Chang CY (1976). Heavy-particle therapy in acromegaly and Cushing disease. JAMA 235: 2307-2310.

57. Lawrence JH, Tobias CA, Chong C (1978). The treatment of pituitary neoplasma with heavy particles. In: Fahlbusch R, Von Werder K (eds). Treatment of pituitary adenomas. Stuttgart: Thieme Verlag, pp 266-272.
58. Liuzzi A, Chiodini PG, Botalla L, Sivestrini F, Müller EE (1974). Growth hormone (GH)-releasing activity of TRH and GH-lowering effect of dopaminergic drugs in acromegaly: homogeneity in the two responses. J Clin Endocrinol Metab 39: 871-876.
59. Camanni F, Massara F, Belforte LK, Molinatti GM (1975). Changes in plasma growth hormone levels in normal and acromegalic subjects following administration of 2-bromo-alpha-ergocriptine. J Clin Endocrinol Metab 40: 363-366.
60. Boyd AE, Lebovitz HE, Pfeiffer JB (1970). Stimulation of human growth hormone secretion by L-dopa. N Engl J Med 283: 1425-1429.
61. Faglia G, Beck-Peccoz P, Travaglini P, Paracchi A, Spada A, Lewin A (1973). Elevations in plasma growth hormone concentration after luteinizing hormone releasing hormone (LRH) in patients with active acromegaly. J Clin Endocrinol Metab 37: 338-340.
62. Chikara K, Kaji H, Minimitani N, Kodoma H, Kita T, Goto B, Chiba T, Coy DH, Fujita T (1984). Stimulation of growth hormone by vaso-active intestinal polypeptide in acromegaly. J Clin Endocrinol Metab 58: 81-86.
63. Pieters GFFM, Hermus ARMM, Smals AGH, Kloppenborg PWC (1984). Paradoxical responsiveness of growth hormone to corticotrophin-releasing factor in acromegaly. J Clin Endocrinol Metab 58: 560-562.
64. Thorner MO, Chait A, Aitken M, Benker G, Bloom SR, Mortimer CH, Sanders P, Stuart-Masson A, Besser GM (1975). Bromocriptine treatment of acromegaly. Br Med J 1: 299-303.
65. Sachdev Y, Tunbridge WMG, Weightman DR, Gomez-Pan A, Duns A, Hall R (1975). Bromocriptine treatment in acromegaly. Lancet 2: 1164-1168.
66. Summers VK, Hipklin LJ, Diver MJ, Davis JC (1975). Treatment of acromegaly with bromocriptine. J Clin Endocrinol Metab 40: 904-906.
67. Dunn PJ, Donald RA, Espiner EA (1977). Bromocriptine suppression of plasma growth hormone in acromegaly. Clin Endocrinol (Oxf) 7: 272-281.
68. Belforte L, Camanni F, Chiodini PG, Liuzzi A, Massara F, Molinatti GM, Müller EE, Silvestrini F (1977). Long-term treatment with 2-Br-alpha- ergocryptine in acromegaly. Acta Endocrinol (Copenh) 85: 235-248.
69. Schwinn G, Dirks H, McIntosh C, Köbberling J (1977). Metabolic and clinical studies on patients with acromegaly treated with bromocriptine over 22 months. Eur J Clin Invest 7: 101-107.
70. Wass JAH, Thorner MO, Morris DV, Rees LH, Stuart-Mason A, Jones AE, Besser GM (1977). Long-term treatment of acromegaly with bromocriptine. Br Med J 1: 875-878.
71. Roelfsema F, Goslings BM, Frölich M, Moolenaar AJ, Van Seters AP, Van Slooten H (1979). The influence of bromocriptine on serum levels of growth hormone and other pituitary hormones and its metabolic effects in active acromegaly. Clin Endocrinol (Oxf) 11: 235-244.
72. Pelkonen R, Ylikahri R, Karonen SL (1980). Bromocriptine treatment of patients with acromegaly resistant to conventional therapy. Clin Endocrinol (Oxf) 12: 219-224.
73. Lindholm J. Riishede J, Vestergaard S, Hummer L, Faber O, Hogen C (1981). No effect of bromocriptine in acromegaly: a controlled trial. N Engl J Med 304: 1450-1454.
74. Wass JAH, Clemmons DR, Underwood LE, Barrow I, Besser JM, Van Wyk JJ (1982). Changes in circulating somatomedin-C levels in bromocriptine treated acromegaly. Clin Endocrinol (Oxf) 17: 369-377.
75. Thorner MO, Besser GM, Wass JAH, Liuzzi A, Hall R, Müller EE, Chiodini PG (1981). Bromocriptine in acromegaly. N Engl J Med 305: 1092-1093.
76. Halse J, Haugen HN, Bohner T (1977). Bromocriptine treatment in acromegaly: clinical and biochemical effects. Acta Endocrinol (Copenh) 86: 464-472.

77. Lundin L. Liunghall S, Wide L, Bostrum J (1978). Bromocriptine therapy in eleven patients with acromegaly. Acta Endocrinol (Copenh) 88, suppl 216: 207-216.
78. Brooks AP, Stephen PJ, Nairu IM, Strong JA (1979). Bromocriptine and acromegaly: therapeutic implications. J Royal Soc Med 72: 562-564.
79. Maneschi F (1980). Reappraisal of bromocriptine treatment for acromegaly. Horm Res 12: 191-205.
80. Lamberts SWJ, Liuzzi A, Chiodini PG, Verde S, Klijn JGM, Birkenhäger JC (1982). The value of prolactin levels in the prediction of the responsiveness of growth hormone secretion to bromocriptine and TRH in acromegaly. Eur J Clin Invest 12: 151-155.
81. Lamberts SWJ, Klijn JGM, van Vroonhoven CGJ, Stefano SZ, Liuzzi A (1983). The role of prolactin in the inhibitory action of bromocriptine on growth hormone secretion in acromegaly. Acta Endocrinol (Copenh) 103: 446-450.
82. Moriondi P, Travaglini P, Rondena M, Beck Peccoz P, Contin Puglisi F, Ambrosi B, Faglia G (1980). Prolactin secretion in acromegaly. In: Faglia G, Giovanelli MA, Macleod RM (eds). Pituitary microadenomas. London, New York: Academic Press: pp247-255.
83. Nieuwenhuijzen Kruseman AC, Bots GThAM, Roelfsema F, Frölich M, van Dulken H (1983). Immunocytochemical growth hormone and prolactin in pituitary adenomas causing acromegaly and their relationship to basal serum hormone levels and the growth hormone response to thyrotropin releasing hormone. Clin Endocrinol (Oxf) 19: 1-8.
84. Oppizzi G, Botalla L, Verde G, Cozzi R, Liuzzi A, Chiodini PG (1980). Homogeneity in the growth hormone-lowering effect of dopamine and somatostatin in acromegaly. J Clin Endocrinol Metab 51: 616-619.
85. Liuzzi A, Chiodini PG, Silvestrini F, Cozzi R, Oppizzi G, Botalla L, Verde G (1980). Effects of neuroactive drugs on growth hormone and prolactin secretion in acromegaly. In: Faglia G, Giovanelli MA, Macleod RM (eds). Pituitary microadenomas. London, New York: Academic Press: pp 367-382.
86. Carmina E, Lo Coco R, Lanzara P, Janni A (1979). Effect of the acute administration of haloperidol and pimozide on plasma GH-levels in acromegaly. Acta Endocrinol (Copenh) 91: 609-615.

CHAPTER II

Plasma growth hormone suppressive effect of bromocriptine in acromegaly. Evaluation by plasma GH day profiles and plasma GH concentrations during oral glucose tolerance tests

J.W.R. Nortier, R.J.M. Croughs, J.H.H. Thijssen and F. Schwarz

Department of Endocrinology, University Hospital, State University of Utrecht, 3500 CG Utrecht, The Netherlands

SUMMARY

In most studies reporting favourable results of chronic bromocriptine treatment in acromegaly, plasma GH levels are measured at fixed intervals during the day. Negative results are reported in one major study measuring plasma GH levels during oral glucose tolerance tests (Lindholm et al., 1981). This study does not mention the time interval between the last dose of bromocriptine and the performance of an OGTT, but due to the short duration of action of bromocriptine this may be critical. Therefore, in the present report the plasma GH suppressive effect of bromocriptine in acromegaly is studied using plasma GH day-profiles as well as OGTT's during continued bromocriptine administration and OGTT's at two different time intervals after the last dose of bromocriptine. Twelve patients with clinically active acromegaly were treated with 10-20 mg bromocriptine for 6-9 months. After 6-9 months during continued bromocriptine administration the plasma GH suppressive effect of bromocriptine was evaluated by the mean of four plasma GH determinations during the day and by the mean of seven plasma GH determinations during oral glucose tolerance tests (OGTT's) performed 1 h, 10 h and 34 h after the last dose. The percentage decrease of the mean plasma GH level during the day induced by chronic bromocriptine treatment showed a good correlation ($r = 0.86$, $p < 0.001$) with the percentage decrease of the mean plasma GH level during OGTT, if the post-treatment test was carried out one hour after the last dose of bromocriptine. When OGTT was performed 10 h after the last dose no significant correlation ($r = 0.17$) was found and after 34 h a rebound of the mean plasma GH level occurred in eight patients. It is

Clinical Endocrinology (1984), 20, 565-571.

concluded that measurement of the mean plasma GH level during the day or during OGTT are equally effective indicators of the suppressive effect of bromocriptine treatment on GH secretion in acromegaly if the OGTT is performed 1 h after the last dose of bromocriptine.

INTRODUCTION

Since 1974 the dopamine agonist bromocriptine has been used in the medical treatment of acromegaly. Good results with regard to plasma GH suppression and to clinical efficacy have been reported by a number of investigators (Thorner et al., 1975; Sachdev et al., 1975; Wass et al., 1977; Belforte et al., 1977; Pelkonen et al., 1980, Wass et al., 1982).

In most of these studies results of treatment were evaluated by measuring plasma GH levels at fixed intervals during the day during continued bromocriptine administration. Negative results were reported in a recent multicentre double-blind cross-over study (Lindholm et al., 1981) and in two earlier studies (Summers et al., 1975; Dunn et al., 1977). Since in these studies results of treatment were evaluated by measuring plasma GH levels during oral glucose tolerance tests (OGTT's) or only during 6 h of the day, these discrepancies might be due to differences in techniques of evaluation. On the other hand bromocriptine has a short duration of action; thus the time interval between the last dose of bromocriptine and the performance of an OGTT may be critical.

We therefore decided to study the plasma GH suppressive effect of bromocriptine in a limited number of acromegalic patients using plasma GH day-profiles as well as OGTT's during continued bromocriptine administration and OGTT's at two different time intervals after the last dose of bromocriptine.

PATIENTS AND METHODS

Patients

The study was carried out on twelve acromegalic patients. Six had been treated with external irradiation, two with surgery, two with both surgery and external irradiation, two had not received any treatment at the time of the present study. The median interval between external irradiation and the beginning of bromocriptine therapy was 5.5 years (range 3-21 years). Four patients had partial or complete pituitary insufficiency; all received appropriate hormonal replacement (Table 1). PRL levels were elevated in five patients. They were selected at random from a larger group of acromegalic

Table 1. Patient data

Patient no.	Age (yrs)	Sex	Previous therapy[1]	Pituitary hormone deficiency	Basal GH[2] (mU/l)	Bromocriptine therapy	
						Dose (mg)	Duration (months)
1	51	F	Irr, 1974		207	10	6
2	33	M	Irr, 1976		53	20	9
3	75	F	None		48	10	6
4	37	M	TFS, Irr, 1979	FSH, LH	43	20	9
5	65	M	Irr, 1961		28	20	9
6	51	M	Irr, 1977	FSH, LH	15	10	6
7	67	F	TSS, 1964	ACTH, TSH LH, FSH	33	10	6
8	55	M	TSS, 1964		30	20	9
9	52	F	TFS, 1960 Irr, 1971	TSH	20	20	9
10	55	F	Irr, 1976		17	20	9
11	58	M	None		13	20	9
12	41	F	Irr, 1978		11	20	9

[1] TSS, transsphenoidal surgery; TFS, transfrontal surgery; Irr, external irradiation.
[2] Mean of four determinations at 08.30 h (fasting), 13.00 h, 17.00 h and 19.00 h.

patients who were all treated with bromocriptine for 6-9 months (Nortier et al., 1983).

Bromocriptine treatment

All patients were treated with bromocriptine 10 mg daily in four divided doses. This treatment was continued for a period of six months in those patients showing a decrease of the mean basal plasma GH level of at least 50%. In the other patients the dose was increased to 20 mg daily after three months and continued for a further period of six months.

Plasma GH profiles

Day-profiles (obtained by measuring GH levels at 0830 h, fasting, 1300 h, 1700 h and 1900 h) were performed in all patients before bromocriptine treatment and were repeated after six months in the patients treated with 10 mg bromocriptine and after nine months in the patients treated with 20 mg bromocriptine. These day- profiles were obtained during continued bromocriptine treatment.

Plasma GH levels during OGTT's

The tests were performed in all patients before bromocriptine treatment and were repeated after six months in the patients treated with 10 mg bromocriptine and after nine months in the patients treated with 20 mg bromocriptine. After a 75 g glucose load plasma GH levels were measured at 0, 15, 30, 60, 90, 120 and 150 min. On separate days OGTT's were performed during bromocriptine treatment (1 h after the last dose), after an over-night fast (10 h after the last dose) and 1 d after bromocriptine withdrawal (34 h after the last dose).

Plasma GH assay

GH (1 µg/l = 2 mU/l) was determined by radioimmunoassay using the SORIN kit (Sorin Biomedica, Saluggia, Italy) with a standard calibrated with the first International Reference preparation (MRC 66/217). The lower limit of detection was approximately 1 mU/l. Intra- and inter-assay variations were 6 and 7.9% ($n = 31$) respectively.

RESULTS

Table 2 summarizes the effect of chronic bromocriptine treatment on plasma GH day-profiles and plasma GH levels during OGTT's. The plasma GH levels during OGTT before and during bromocriptine treatment respectively 1, 10 and 34 hours after the last dose of bromocriptine are depicted in Fig. 1. Chronic bromocriptine therapy induced a reduction of mean plasma GH levels by at least 50% of the initial values in eight patients. The percentage decrease of mean plasma GH level during the day induced by chronic bromocriptine treatment showed a good relation ($r = 0.86$, $p < 0.001$) with the percentage decrease of the mean plasma GH level during OGTT, if the post-treatment test was carried out 1 h after the last dose of bromocriptine (Table 2, Fig. 2-A). No significant correlation ($r = 0.17$) was found if the post-treatment OGTT was carried out 10 h after the last dose of bromocriptine (Table 2, Fig. 2-B). When OGTT's were carried out 34 h after the last dose of bromocriptine, a rebound increase of the mean plasma GH level was found in eight patients (Table 2, Fig. 1). An increase of the mean plasma GH level during OGTT of at least 184% was found in patients 1-6, five of whom had basal plasma GH levels of at least 28 mU/l, and also five of these patients showed a reduction of the mean plasma GH level during the day by more than 50% as a consequence of chronic bromocriptine treatment. Thus in most patients with high basal plasma GH levels and with effective reduction of the plasma GH level during bromocriptine therapy hypersecretion of GH after discontinuation of the drug seems to occur.

Table 2. Effect of chronic bromocriptine treatment on plasma GH day-profiles and on plasma GH levels during OGTT's

Patient no.	Mean plasma GH (mU/l) during the day			Mean plasma GH (mU/l) during OGTT						
	B[1] (range)	D[2] (range)	Δ GH (%)	B[1]	D[2] 1 h[3]	Δ GH (%)	D[2] 10 h[4]	Δ GH (%)	D[2] 34 h[5]	Δ GH (%)
1	207 (170–260)	9 (5–12)	-96	175	26	-85	3	-98	557	+218
2	53 (44– 60)	18 (16–22)	-66	48	28	-42	26	-46	149	+210
3	48 (28– 61)	21 (15–34)	-56	31	13	-58	21	-32	88	+184
4	43 (39– 48)	38 (32–43)	-12	42	29	-31	18	-58	146	+248
5	28 (19– 38)	8 (5–12)	-72	25	9	-64	40	+60	96	+284
6	15 (14– 18)	4 (4– 4)	-73	11	5	-55	4	-64	70	+536
7	33 (21– 53)	8 (5–16)	-76	23	6	-74	19	-17	21	-9
8	30 (16– 51)	28 (14–35)	-7	30	37	+23	28	-7	55	+83
9	20 (17– 23)	10 (7–12)	-50	15	8	-46	9	-40	15	0
10	17 (11– 21)	10 (9–12)	-41	13	9	-31	11	-15	11	-15
11	13 (9– 15)	7 (5– 9)	-46	15	7	-53	9	-40	19	+27
12	11 (9– 14)	5 (3– 8)	-55	15	6	-60	5	-67	9	-40
Mean change (± SEM)			-53 ± 7.4			-48 ± 7.9		-35 ± 11.3		+144 ± 48.9

[1] B, before bromocriptine treatment.
[2] D, during bromocriptine treatment.
[3] 1 h, OGTT performed 1 h after the last dose of bromocriptine.
[4] 10 h, OGTT performed 10 h after the last dose of bromocriptine.
[5] 34 h, OGTT performed 34 h after the last dose of bromocriptine.

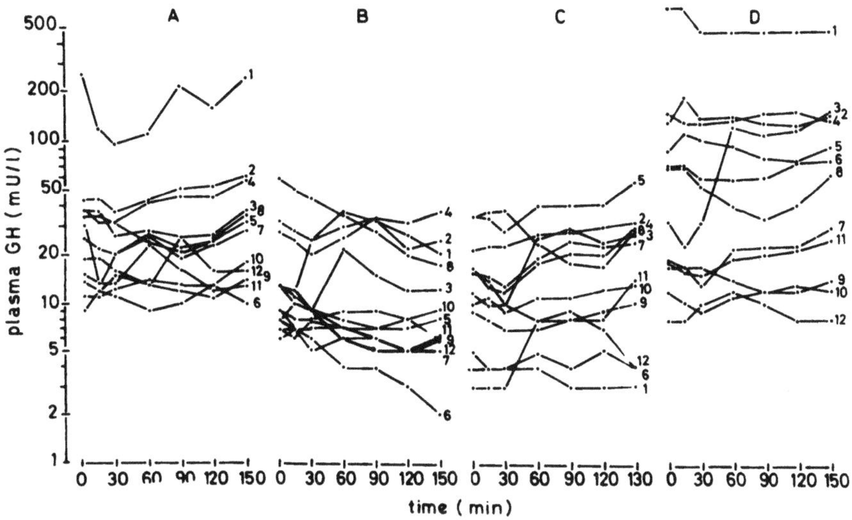

Fig. 1. Individual plasma GH levels after oral glucose loading **A**, before bromocriptine therapy; **B**, during chronic bromocriptine therapy 1 h after the last dose; **C**, 10 h after the last dose and **D**, 34 h after the last dose.

Fig. 2. **A**, correlation between the percentage change of the mean plasma GH level during the day (horizontal axis) and the mean plasma GH level during OGTT performed 1 h after the last dose of bromocriptine (vertical axis); **B**, correlation between the percentage change of the mean plasma GH level during the day (horizontal axis) and the mean plasma GH level during OGTT performed 10 h after the last dose of bromocriptine (vertical axis).

DISCUSSION

The present study confirms that chronic bromocriptine treatment effectively reduces plasma GH levels in the majority of patients with acromegaly. Measurement of plasma GH day-profiles and measurement of plasma GH concentrations during OGTT are equally effective indicators of the suppressive effect of bromocriptine treatment on the GH secretion if OGTT's are performed 1 h after the last dose of bromocriptine. OGTT's may give misleading results if they are carried out before the morning dose of bromocriptine has been administered. Due to a rebound release of GH this is *a fortiori* the case if OGTT's are performed one day after interruption of bromocriptine treatment.

Some studies have reported negative results of chronic bromocriptine treatment in acromegaly. Summers et al. (1975) reported no effect in 7 of 8 patients. GH responsiveness to bromocriptine was evaluated by OGTT's during continued bromocriptine treatment 2 h after the last dose of bromocriptine. However, these authors used rather low doses of bromocriptine (2.5 mg every 8 h) for a period of only 4 to 5 weeks. Dunn et al. (1977) found no effect of 20 mg bromocriptine given during a 3 month period in 3 of 5 acromegalic patients. Although bromocriptine was continued throughout the test-day at the end of the 3 month period, plasma GH levels were only measured hourly for 6 hours in 4 patients and only at 1000 h in the morning in one patient.

Lindholm et al. (1981) evaluated the effect of bromocriptine treatment in acromegaly using OGTT's. The negative results of this study have been criticized (Thorner et al., 1981), as the interval between the initiation of the OGTT and the last administered dose of bromocriptine is not mentioned. This information is the more important as our study shows that a rebound release of GH is found particularly in those cases responding to chronic bromocriptine treatment with a reduction of plasma GH levels of more than 50%, although a rebound was also present in two patients who showed a reduction of plasma GH levels of less than 15%. This phenomenon has been observed previously (Belforte et al., 1977; Feek et al., 1981) and is probably related to inhibition of GH release, whereas GH synthesis is not impaired. In agreement with this hypothesis is the observation that a direct stimulus to GH release such as TRH is not inhibited by bromocriptine (Ishibashi et al., 1977).

Thorner et al.(1981) also criticized the use of OGTT's to evaluate the results of chronic bromocriptine treatment as physiological control of GH secretion is not tested. However, our study shows that if bromocriptine treatment is continued both GH day- profiles and plasma GH levels during OGTT's are equally useful indicators of the GH suppressive effect of bromocriptine treatment in acromegaly.

REFERENCES

Belforte, L., Camanni, F., Chiodini, P.G., Liuzzi, A., Massara, F., Molinatti, G.M., Müller, E.E. & Silvestrini, F. (1977). Long-term treatment with 2-Br-alpha-ergocryptine in acromegaly. Acta Endocrinologica, 85, 235-248.

Dunn, P.J., Donals, R.A. & Espiner, E.A. (1977). Bromocriptine suppression of plasma growth hormone in acromegaly. Clinical Endocrinology, 7, 273-281.

Feek, G.M., Bevan, J.S., Taylor, S., Brown, N.S. & Baird, J.D. (1981). The effect of bromocriptine on insulin secretion and glucose tolerance in patients with acromegaly. Clinical Endocrinology, 15, 473-478.

Ishibashi, M., Yamaji, T. & Kosaka, K. (1977). Effect of bromoergocryptine on TRH-induced growth hormone and prolactin release in acromegalic patients. Journal of Clinical Endocrinology and Metabolism, 45, 275-279.

Lindholm, J., Riishede, J., Vestergaard, S., Hummer, L., Faber, O. & Hagen, C. (1981). No effect of bromocriptine in acromegaly: a controlled trial. New England Journal of Medicine, 304, 1450-1454.

Nortier, J.W.R., Croughs, R.J.M., Thijssen, J.H.H. & Schwarz, F. (1983). Changes in plasma growth hormone levels and clinical activity in bromocriptine treated acromegaly resistant to conventional therapy. European Journal of Clinical Investigation, 13, 2, part II, 33 (abstract).

Pelkonen, R., Ylikahri, R. & Karonen, S.L. (1980). Bromocriptine treatment of patients with acromegaly resistant to conventional therapy. Clinical Endocrinology, 12, 219-224.

Sachdev, Y., Tunbridge, W.M.G., Weightman, D.R., Gomez-Pan, A. & Hall, R. (1975). Bromocriptine therapy in acromegaly. Lancet, ii, 1164-1168.

Summers, V.K., Hipkin, L.J., Diver, M.J. & Davis, J.C. (1975). Treatment of acromegaly with bromocriptine. Journal of Clinical Endocrinology and Metabolism, 40, 904-906.

Thorner, M.O., Chait, A., Aitken, M., Benker, G., Bloom, S.R., Mortimer, C.H., Sanders, P., Stuart Mason, A. & Besser, G.M. (1975). Bromocriptine treatment of acromegaly. British Medical Journal, i, 299-303.

Thorner, M.O., Besser, G.M., Wass, J.A.H., Liuzzi, A., Hall, R., Müller, E.E. & Chiodini, P.G. (1981). Bromocriptine in acromegaly. New England Journal of Medicine, 305, 1092-1093.

Wass, J.A.H., Thorner, M.O., Morris, D.V., Rees, L.H., Stuart-Mason, A., Jones, A.E. & Besser, G.M. (1977). Long-term treatment of acromegaly with bromocriptine. British Medical Journal, i, 875-878.

Wass, J.A.H., Clemmons, D.R., Underwood, L.E., Barrow, I., Besser, G.M., & van Wyk, J.L. (1982). Changes in circulating somatomedin-C levels in bromocriptine treated acromegaly. Clinical Endocrinology, 17, 369-377.

CHAPTER III

Changes in plasma GH levels and clinical activity during bromocriptine therapy in acromegaly. The value of predictive tests

J.W.R. Nortier, R.J.M. Croughs, G.H. Donker, J.H.H. Thijssen, and F. Schwarz

Department of Endocrinology, State University of Utrecht, Catharijnesingel 101, Utrecht, The Netherlands

ABSTRACT

Twenty-seven patients with active acromegaly despite previous treatment by surgery and/or radiotherapy received bromocriptine in a dose of 10-20 mg daily for a period of 6-9 months. The results of chronic bromocriptine treatment were evaluated by measurement of plasma growth hormone (GH) levels during the day and by subjective and objective criteria of clinical activity. The results of chronic bromocriptine treatment were also compared with four biochemical criteria obtained before treatment e.g. basal plasma prolactin (Prl) levels and the plasma GH response to oral administration of 2.5 mg bromocriptine respectively iv administration of 200 µg TRH and 500 µg somatostatin. The main observations may be summarized as follows: 1) The mean pre-treatment GH levels during the day ranged from 6-207 mU/l. Hyperprolactinaemia was present in 6 patients. 2) During bromocriptine treatment mean plasma GH levels decreased to less than 50% in 11 patients (GH responders) whereas in 19 patients changes of mean plasma GH levels and of subjective criteria of clinical activity were concordant. 3) Glucose tolerance improved significantly ($p < 0.01$) in 10 GH-responders and the urinary hydroxyproline/creatinine ratio decreased significantly ($p < 0.05$) in 8 GH-responders. 4) Five out of 6 patients with hyperprolactinaemia belonged to the group of GH-responders. 5) A single dose of 2.5 mg bromocriptine induced a more than 50% decrease of plasma GH in 8 of 11 GH-responders and in 5 of 16 GH non-responders. 6) The iv injection of 200 µg TRH was followed by a rise of plasma GH of more than 100% in 9 of 11 GH-responders and in 6 of 16 non-responders. 7) Responsiveness to both a single dose of bromocriptine and TRH was found in 8 of 11 GH-responders and in 3 of 16 GH non-responders.

Acta Endocrinologica 1984, 106, 175-183

Conclusions

1. Bromocriptine is effective as adjunctive therapy when active acromegaly persists after treatment with surgery and/or radiotherapy.
2. In general, a good correlation is found between GH responsiveness and subjective and objective criteria of clinical activity during bromocriptine treatment.
3. Hyperprolactinaemia predicts GH responsiveness to chronic bromocriptine treatment with high specificity.
4. The combination of a bromocriptine test and TRH test are of best predictive value with respect to the results of chronic bromocriptine therapy in normoprolactinaemic acromegalics.

INTRODUCTION

Early transsphenoidal surgery with the aim of selective adenomectomy is the most effective treatment in patients with acromegaly, particularly in smaller tumours and when GH levels are below 100 mU/l (Quabbe 1982). However, the cure rate of acromegaly by microsurgery is still low despite improved surgical techniques (Faglia et al. 1978; Arafah et al. 1980; Jaquet et al. 1980; Hulting et al. 1982). The response to external irradiation is often slow in onset and may still occur after 5-10 years (Eastman et al. 1979).

Therefore the possibility of additional medical treatment with the dopamine agonist bromocriptine has raised great interest. In most studies favourable responses to bromocriptine therapy have been reported in 50-80% of patients (Thorner et al. 1975; Sachdev et al. 1975; Wass et al. 1977; Belforte et al. 1977; Schwinn et al. 1977). In some studies results have been disappointing (Summers et al. 1975; Dunn et al. 1977; Cassar et al. 1977; Roelfsema et al. 1979; Lindholm et al. 1981), in others favourable results have only been observed if the initial plasma GH levels were moderately elevated (Pelkonen et al. 1980; Quabbe 1982). Moreover, the criteria used in these studies to define the clinical and plasma GH response to bromocriptine are not uniform. Discrepancies between the degree of clinical improvement and the reduction in circulating plasma GH levels have been noted frequently (Wass et al. 1977; Halse et al. 1977; Lundin et al. 1978; Brooks et al. 1979; Maneschi 1980).

Acromegalic patients who show a reduction of the plasma GH level of more than 50% in an acute suppression test with 2.5 mg bromocriptine, frequently also show a more than 50% reduction of the plasma GH level during chronic bromocriptine treatment (Belforte et al. 1977; Schwinn et al. 1977; Roelfsema et al. 1979). These patients are also often characterized by a rise of the plasma GH level after administration of TRH (Liuzzi et al. 1974;

Schwinn et al. 1977; Roelfsema et al. 1979), a more than 50% decrease of the plasma GH level during somatostatin infusion (Oppizzi et al. 1980) and elevated basal prolactin levels (Lamberts et al. 1982). No investigations are reported in which these criteria were determined in the same group of patients and subsequently compared with the results of chronic bromocriptine therapy.

The objective of the present study was to compare the plasma GH response to chronic bromocriptine therapy with subjective and objective criteria of clinical activity in patients with acromegaly still active after surgery and/or radiotherapy; furthermore to assess the predictive value with respect to the results of long-term bromocriptine therapy of changes of plasma GH after a single dose of 2.5 mg bromocriptine, after TRH, during somatostatin infusion and of the basal prolactin level.

PATIENTS AND METHODS

The study was carried out on 27 acromegalic patients. They all showed clinical activity with failure to suppress plasma GH levels to less than 4 mU/l after a 75 g glucose load. Sixteen patients had been treated with external irradiation, 7 with surgery, 4 with both surgery and radiotherapy. Eleven patients had partial or complete pituitary insufficiency; all received appropriate hormonal replacement (Table 1).

Regimen of bromocriptine

The patients were treated with bromocriptine 10 mg daily in four divided doses. This treatment was continued for a period of 6 months in patients showing a decrease of the mean plasma GH level of at least 50%. In the other patients the dose was increased to 20 mg daily after 3 months and continued for a further period of 6 months.

Subjective criteria of clinical activity

Before and during continued bromocriptine therapy after 6-9 months an assessment was made of acromegalic symptoms by a clinical score of maximal 14 points. This score was obtained by adding the scores for each symptom according to the degree of severity in the following way: acral swelling 0-3 points, hyperhidrosis 0-2 points, headache 0-2 points, weakness-/fatigue 0-2 points, paraesthesia 0-1 point, sleep-apnoe 0-1 point, sexual insufficiency 0-1 point, hirsutism/hypertrichosis 0-1 point, joint/muscle pain 0-1 point. Patients who showed a reduction of this score of more than 50% were arbitrarily defined as 'symptomatic responders'.

Table 1. Patient data

Patient no.	Age yrs	Sex	Previous therapy[1]	Pituitary hormone deficiency	Basal GH[2] mU/l	Basal Prl[3] U/l
1. Sle	50	F	Irr, 1974		207	0.23
2. Ros	48	M	TSS, 1971	ACTH, TSH, LH, FSH	122	0.05
3. Boo	65	M	TSS, 1965	ACTH, TSH, LH, FSH	72	0.74
4. Lok	41	M	TSS, 1971	ACTH, LH, FSH	59	0.08
5. Vle	32	M	Irr, 1976		52	0.46
6. Zie	41	F	Irr, 1965		47	0.25
7. Bee	36	M	TSS, 1979 Irr, 1979	LH, FSH	43	2.25
8. Pel	35	M	TSS, 1966 TFS, 1969 Irr, 1969	ACTH, TSH, LH, FSH	40	0.05
9. Ven	37	F	Irr, 1975		38	1.8
10. Nob	66	F	TSS, 1964	ACTH, TSH, LH, FSH	33	0.45
11. Bri	54	M	TSS, 1964		30	0.11
12. Kip	65	M	Irr, 1977		29	0.27
13. Kel	65	M	Irr, 1961		28	0.84
14. Tan	44	M	Irr, 1980	ACTH, TSH, LH, FSH	28	0.52
15. Jan	47	F	TFS, 1967	ACTH, LH, FSH	24	0.37
16. Jac	37	F	Irr, 1975		23	0.58
17. Swa	51	F	TFS, 1960 Irr, 1970	TSH	20	1.57
18. Beu	31	F	Irr, 1977		20	0.44
19. Lel	52	M	Irr, 1979		16	0.48
20. Mas	54	F	Irr, 1976		17	0.28
21. Vla	50	M	Irr, 1977	FSH, LH	15	2.75
22. Aup	57	F	TSS, 1970		14	0.31
23. Goe	45	F	Irr, 1979		14	0.59
24. Pal	41	F	Irr, 1978		11	0.21
25. Age	71	F	Irr, 1954		7	0.32
26. Wie	31	F	TFS, 1977 Irr, 1977	ACTH, TSH, LH, FSH	6	0.23
27. Eek	35	M	Irr, 1976		6	0.13

[1] TSS, transsphenoidal surgery; TFS, transfrontal surgery; Irr, external irradiation.
[2] Mean of 4 determinations during the day.
[3] Mean of 3 determinations on separate days (fasting).
Substitutional therapy: ACTH deficiency, cortisone-acetate 25 mg at 08.00 h, 12.5 mg at 18.00 h; TSH deficiency, 100– 250 μg L-thyroxine daily; LH, FSH deficiency, female: cyclic 25 μg ethinyl-oestradiol and male: 250 mg testosterone im 3-weekly.

Objective criteria of clinical activity

Before and during continued bromocriptine therapy the following assessments were made:

- After overnight fasting glucose tolerance was assessed by measuring blood glucose levels during 150 min after a 75 g glucose load.

The area under the glucose curve was estimated by summating 7 blood glucose samples obtained at 0, 15, 30, 60, 90 , 120 and 150 min.
- Hydroxyproline excretion (expressed as the hydroxyproline/creatinine ratio) was measured from 24 h urine collections.
- Measurement of the mean circumference of the fourth and fifth finger of both hands using a set of jeweller's rings.

Plasma GH levels

Mean plasma GH levels, obtained by averaging plasma GH levels at 08.30 h (fasting), 13.00, 17.00 and 19.00 h, were determined in all patients before bromocriptine treatment and were repeated after 6 months in the patients treated with 10 mg bromocriptine and after 9 months in those treated with 20 mg bromocriptine during continued bromocriptine therapy. The mean value during the day was used as the index of GH secretion before and during bromocriptine therapy. Patients who showed a reduction of the mean plasma GH levels during the day of more than 50% were arbitrarily defined as 'GH-responders'.

Predictive tests

Before bromocriptine therapy was started the following tests were performed on separate days with measurement of plasma GH at the times indicated:
- TRH test; 200 µg TRH was administered iv; blood samples were taken at -15, 0, 20 and 60 min.
- Acute bromocriptine suppression test; 2.5 mg bromocriptine was administered orally; blood samples were taken at -15, 0, 120, 240, 360 and 480 min.
- Somatostatin suppression test; 500 µg somatostatin was administered iv during 1 h; blood samples were taken at -15, 0, 20, 60 and 120 min.
- Basal Prl level; this was obtained by averaging three fasting levels at 08.30 h taken on separate days.

Assay methods

Blood sugar was measured with the hexokinase method using a Technicon Autoanalyzer II. All determinations were done in duplicate.

Plasma GH was determined by radioimmunoassay (1 µg/l = 2 mU/l) using the Sorin kit (Sorin Biomedica, Saluggia, Italy) with a standard calibrated on the first international Reference Preparation (MRC 66/217). The sensitivity was approximately 1 mU/l; intra- and inter-assay variations were 6 and 7.9% (n = 31) respectively.

Prl was measured by radioimmunoassay (commercial IRE-kit). The intra-

and inter-assay variations were 7 and 11%, respectively. The values are expressed as U/l (25 ng/ml = 1 IU/l MRC 71/222). Normal basal values in our laboratory are < 0.6 U/l in females and < 0.5 U/l in males.

Hydroxyproline was measured as described by Firschein & Schill (1966).

RESULTS

The mean pre-treatment plasma GH levels during the day ranged from 6 to 207 mU/l. The mean of the basal Prl levels before treatment ranged from 0.05 to 2.75 U/l (Table 1). In 6 patients (22%) the plasma Prl level was elevated. In all patients except 1 plasma Prl levels fell to very low levels during chronic bromocriptine treatment (mean 0.04, range 0.01-0.41 U/l). The changes of the mean plasma GH levels and of the clinical scores of symptoms are depicted in Fig.1. In 7 patients a decrease of both the mean plasma GH level and of the score of symptoms of more than 50% was observed (patient no. 1, 9, 10, 13, 18, 21, 24). In 8 other patients the decrease of the mean plasma GH

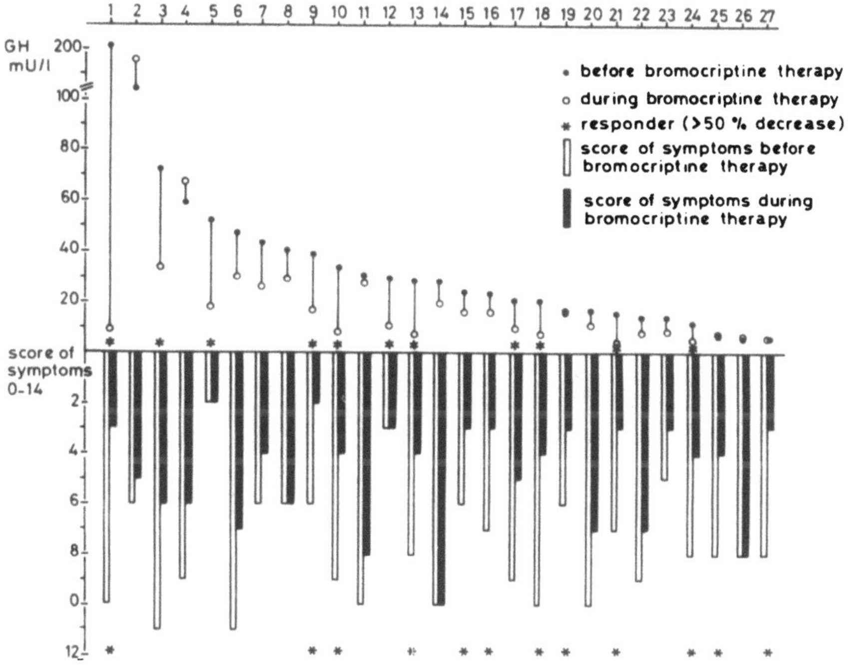

Fig. 1. Mean plasma GH level before (●), and during (○) bromocriptine treatment; clinical score of acromegalic symptoms before (□) and during (■) bromocriptine treatment in 27 acromegalic patients. Asterisks indicate a decrease of more than 50%.

Table 2. The sum of blood glucose values during oral glucose tolerance tests before (B) and during (D) chronic bromocriptine treatment (left panel); urinary hydroxyproline excretion, expressed as the hydroxyproline/creatinine ratio before (B) and during (D) chronic bromocriptine treatment (right panel). Statistical analysis by Wilcoxon-tests

Sum of blood glucose (mmol/l)						Urinary hydroxyproline/creatine ratio					
GH-responders			GH non-responders			GH-responders			GH non-responders		
Patient no.	B	D	Patient no.	B	D	Patient no.	B	D	Patient no.	B	D
1	74.5	55.9	2	81.3	113.1	1	30.8	15.0	2	13.8	8.6
3	40.1	38.8	4	122.8	80.5	3	18.9	28.3	4	23.1	14.3
5	28.9	21	6	37	36.4	5	33.5	16.9	6	19.4	20.5
10	42.7	23.7	7	36.2	37.8	10	66.2	37.6	7		
12	45.9	45.7	8	36.6	39.6	12	12.3	9.6	8	75.4	59.4
13	79.1	62	11	43.1	40.2	13	14.4	9.2	11	24.8	30.6
17	40.5	38.5	14	35.2	30.9				14	43.6	57.2
18	33.9	28.5	15	117.9	134.5				15	71.3	31.7
21	37.3	34.9	16	31.5	33.8	21	16.9	11.3	16		
24	41	35.1	19	49.2	39.3	24	20.7	20.2	19	22.0	25.6
Mean	46.4	38.4	20	33.1	35.1	Mean	26.7	18.5	20	33.1	18.2
± SEM	± 5.3	± 4.1	22	37.5	42.2	± SEM	± 6.2	± 3.5	22	23.7	9.9
P value		< 0.01	23	37.3	30.5	*P* value		< 0.05	23	16.4	32.7
			25	24.7	30.3				25	23.9	10.3
			26	33.5	20.4				26	17.2	22.9
			27	41	29.8				27	21.7	15.6
			Mean	51	49.4				Mean	30.6	25.5
			± SEM	± 7.9	± 8.6				± SEM	± 5.2	± 4.3
			P value		N.S.				*P* value		N.S.

level and of the score of symptoms was between 25 and 50% (patient no. 3, 6, 7, 15, 16, 17, 20, 23). In 1 patient the mean plasma GH level decreased by 36% whereas the score of symptoms decreased by 22% (patient no. 22). In 3 patients both the decrease of the clinical score and of the mean plasma GH level was less than 20% (patient no. 2, 11, 26). Thus, in 19 patients (70%) changes of the mean plasma GH levels and of clinical symptoms were concordant.

Discordant changes were found in 8 patients. In 4 patients the mean plasma GH level decreased by more than 25% (range 28-65%) whereas the score of symptoms did not change at all (patient no. 5, 8, 12, 14). In the other 4 patients the score of symptoms decreased by more than 25% (range 33-62%) whereas the mean plasma GH levels did not fall (patient no. 4, 19, 25, 27).

The sums of blood sugar values during oral glucose tolerance tests and the urinary hydroxyproline values before and during chronic bromocriptine treatment are shown in Table 2. Blood glucose levels decreased significantly ($p < 0.01$) in 10 GH-responders and urinary hydroxyproline excretion decreased significantly in 8 GH-responders ($p < 0.05$). No significant changes were found in respectively 16 and 14 GH non-responders.

The mean change of the fingercircumference of the fourth and fifth finger of both hands is correlated with the plasma GH response to chronic bromocriptine treatment for each individual patient in Fig.2. ($r = 0.33$, n.s.). In all patients except one a decrease was found. The mean decrease in the GH-responder group was 3 mm, in the GH non-responder group 1.8 mm.

The results of the plasma GH-response to the administration of a single dose of 2.5 mg bromocriptine, 200 µg TRH and 500 µg somatostatin, the basal plasma Prl level and the combination of the responses to TRH and bromocriptine are shown in Table 3 on separate columns for GH-responders and GH non-responders. In all GH-responders one of the four predictive tests was positive, but this was also found in 11 of 16 GH non-responders. All patients with hyperprolactinaemia showed a decrease of more than 50% of the plasma GH level after administration of a single dose of bromocriptine and a rise of more than 100% after administration of TRH. Among the 13 patients who responded to a single dose of bromocriptine, 11 (85%) also responded to TRH. Among 15 patients who responded to TRH, 11 (73%) also responded to a single dose of bromocriptine.

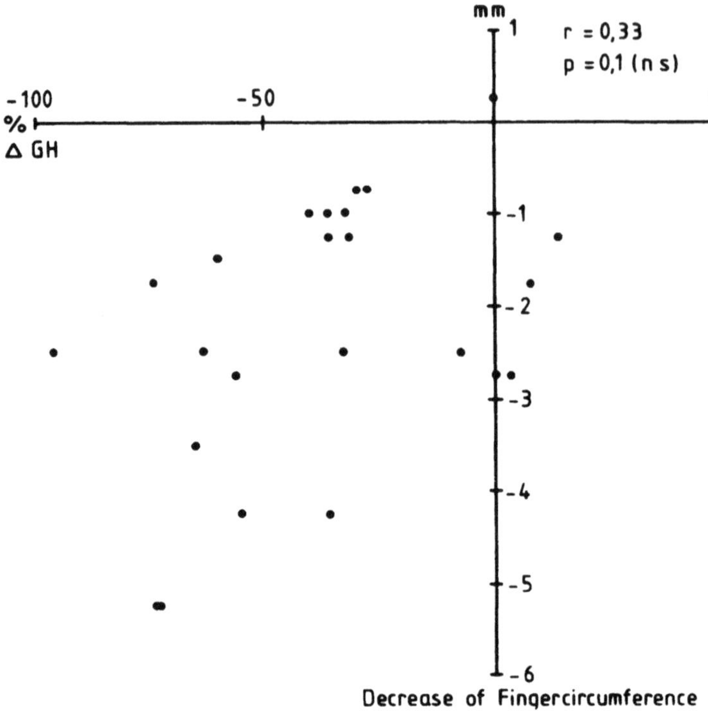

Fig. 2. Correlation between the individual GH response to chronic bromocriptine treatment (horizontal axis) and the change of the mean circumference of the fourth and fifth finger of both hands (vertical axis).

Table 3. The predictive value of four criteria with respect to the results of chronic bromocriptine therapy in 11 GH-responders (A) and 16 GH non-responders (B)

		A	B
I	Acute bromocriptine suppression (more than 50% decrease)	8/11 73%	5/16 31%
II	TRH-GH (more than 100% increase)	9/11 82%	6/16 37%
III	Somatostatin-GH (more than 50% decrease)	8/11 73%	9/16 56%
IV	Hyperprolactinaemia (more than 0.6 U/l)	5/11 45%	1/16 6%
I + II		8/11 73%	3/16 19%

DISCUSSION

Chronic treatment with the dopamine agonist bromocriptine resulted in a considerable subjective and objective clinical improvement as well as in reduction of the plasma GH levels in the majority of this group of patients with acromegaly still active despite treatment by pituitary surgery and/or external irradiation. These findings are in agreement with most studies in which a decrease of the mean plasma GH level during the day of more than 50% has been considered as a positive reponse (Sachdev et al. 1975; Belforte et al. 1977; Schwinn et al. 1977; Wass et al. 1982). Although theoretically in those patients who were irradiated part of the GH suppressive effect of chronic bromocriptine treatment might be due to the external irradiation, it is unlikely that this played an important role as most patients were irradiated more than 3 years before bromocriptine was started and as in most patients plasma GH levels increased to pre-treatment levels after subsequent bromocriptine withdrawal (Nortier et al. 1984, Chapter II).

In 19 of 27 patients (70%) a good correlation was found between changes of the mean plasma GH levels and of symptoms. Discordant changes were found in 8 patients; in 2 of these patients the score of symptoms was low and in 2 other patients the mean plasma GH level was low, making it difficult to find a change. Although a significant improvement was found of glucose tolerance in 10 GH responders and of urinary hydroxyproline excretion in 8 GH responders, discrepancies between these objective criteria of clinical activity and the GH response to chronic bromocriptine therapy were also found, especially among GH non-responders.

Others have found more frequent discrepancies and especially symptomatic improvement out of proportion to the fall in plasma GH (Wass et al. 1977; Halse et al. 1977; Shalet et al. 1980; Marek et al. 1981). Explanations for these discrepancies between the clinical and GH response have been a preferential suppression of the monomeric form of GH ('little GH') which is biologically the most active form (Besser et al. 1976), a change in somatomedin activity (Wass et al. 1982) or a preferential increase in the clearance of monomeric GH by bromocriptine (Maneschi et al. 1978).

Ergot derivatives exert a constrictor action on the capacitance vessels in skin and skeletal muscle (Mellander & Nordenfeld 1976) which could be a factor explaining the lack of correlation between the individual changes of GH and ring size.

A paradoxical decrease of the plasma GH level after administration of L-dopa was described in 17 of 29 acromegalic patients by Liuzzi et al. (1974). In 15 of these patients a paradoxical increase of the plasma GH level after administration of TRH was found as well. Belforte et al. (1977) reported that in 18 of 21 patients who responded to chronic bromocriptine treatment with a decrease of the mean plasma GH level of more than 50%, an acute suppressive effect of a single dose of 2.5 mg bromocriptine was found as well.

The responsiveness of acromegalic adenomas to TRH and/or acute bromocriptine tests has been related to hyperprolactinaemia or to the ability of the adenoma cells to synthesize prolactin (Lamberts et al. 1982, 1983) although this has not been found by others (Moriondo et al. 1980; Nieuwenhuijzen Kruseman et al. 1983).

The increased Prl levels in 6 of our 27 pretreated acromegalic patients were accompanied by responsiveness to TRH and bromocriptine in the acute test in all of them, which is in accordance with the reported studies by Lamberts et al. (1979, 1982, 1983) in untreated acromegalics, although in his last study no correlation was found between the basal Prl level and the TRH response, due to a rather low homogeneity (68%) in responsiveness of GH to TRH and bromocriptine. In addition, in 5 of our 6 hyperprolactinaemic acromegalic patients responsiveness to chronic bromocriptine treatment was found.

A homogeneity in the growth hormone lowering effect of dopamine and somatostatin was reported by Oppizzi et al. (1980) and by Liuzzi et al. (1980). In our patients the degree of inhibition of the plasma GH level during somatostatin infusion gives no additional information as to the chance of success of chronic bromocriptine treatment since the sensitivity (73%) of this test does not differ from the acute bromocriptine suppression test or the TRH test and the specificity is much lower (44%).

In our study acute bromocriptine suppression and a TRH test are of equal value in predicting the plasma GH response to chronic bromocriptine therapy (sensitivity respectively 73 and 82%, specificity respectively 69 and 63%). The combination of the TRH test and the bromocriptine test predicts the response to chronic bromocriptine treatment with the same sensitivity but with higher specificity (81%) than each test separately. All other combinations do not improve the predictive value due to the low specificity of the GH response during somatostatin infusion and to the homogeneity of hyperprolactinaemia and the GH response to TRH and bromocriptine.

REFERENCES

Arafah BM, Brodley S, Kaufman B, Valasso M, Manni A & Pearson O (1980): Transsphenoidal microsurgery in the treatment of acromegaly and gigantism. J Clin Endocrinol Metab 50: 578-585.

Belforte L, Camanni F, Chiodini PG, Liuzzi A, Massara F, Molinatti GM, Müller EE & Silvestrini F (1977): Long-term treatment with 2 Br-alpha-ergocryptine in acromegaly. Acta Endocrinol (Copenh) 85: 235-248.

Besser HGM, Thorner MO, Wass JAH, Jones AE, Lowrey PJ, Rees LH & Jones A (1976): Bromocriptine treatment of acromegaly. Q J Med 45: 695-696.

Brooks AP, Stephan PJ, Nairn IM & Strong JA (1979): Bromocriptine and acromegaly: therapeutic implications. J R Soc Med 72: 562-564.

Cassar J, Mashiter K & Joplin GF (1977): Bromocriptine treatment of acromegaly. Metabolism 26: 539-546.

Dunn PJ, Donald RA & Espiner EA (1977): Bromocriptine suppression of plasma growth hormone in acromegaly. Clin Endocrinol (Oxf) 7: 273-281.

Eastman RC, Gordon P & Roth J (1979): Conventional supervoltage irradiation is an effective treatment for acromegaly. J Clin Endocrinol Metab 48: 931-940.

Faglia G, Paracchi A, Ferrari C & Beck-Peccoz P (1978): Evaluation of the results of transsphenoidal surgery in acromegaly by assessment of the growth hormone response to thyrotropin-releasing hormone. Clin Endocrinol (Oxf) 8: 373-380.

Firschein HE & Schill JP (1966): The determination of total hydroxyproline in urine and bone extracts. Anal Biochem 14: 296-302.

Halse J, Haugen HN & Bohmer T (1977): Bromocriptine treatment in acromegaly: clinical and biochemical effects. Acta Endocrinol (Copenh) 86: 464-472.

Hulting AL, Werner S, Wersäll J, Tribukait B & Anniko M (1982): Normal growth hormone secretion is rare after microsurgical normalization of growth hormone levels in acromegaly. Acta Med Scand 212: 401-405.

Jaquet P, Guibout M, Jaquet C, Grisoli F, Devolx BC, Dumas D & Bert J (1980): Circadian regulation of growth hormone secretion after treatment in acromegaly. J Clin Endocrinol Metab 50: 322-328.

Lamberts SWJ, Klijn JGM, Kwa GH & Birkenhäger JC (1979): The dynamics of growth hormone and prolactin secretion in acromegalic patients with 'mixed' pituitary tumours. Acta Endocrinol (Copenh) 90: 198-210.

Lamberts SWJ, Liuzzi A, Chiodini PG, Verde S, Klijn JGM & Birkenhäger JC (1982): The value of plasma prolactin levels in the prediction of the responsiveness of growth hormone secretion to bromocriptine and TRH in acromegaly. Eur J Clin Invest 12: 151-155.

Lamberts SWJ, Klijn JGM, van Vroonhoven CGH, Stefano SZ & Liuzzi A (1983): The role of prolactin in the inhibitory action of bromocriptine on growth hormone secretion in acromegaly. Acta Endocrinol (Copenh) 103: 446-450.

Lindholm J, Riishede J, Vestergaard S, Hummer L, Faber O & Hagen C (1981): No effect of bromocriptine in acromegaly: a controlled trial. N Engl J Med 304: 1450-1454.

Liuzzi A, Chiodini PG, Botalla L, Silvestrini F & Müller EE (1974): Growth hormone (GH)-releasing activity of TRH and GH-lowering effect of dopaminergic drugs in acromegaly: homogeneity in the two responses. J Clin Endocrinol Metab 39: 871-876.

Liuzzi A, Chiodini PG, Silvestrini F, Cossi R, Oppizzi G, Botalla L & Verde G (1980): Effects of neuroactive drugs on growth hormone and prolactin secretion in acromegaly. In: Faglia G, Giovanelli MA & McLeod RR (eds). Pituitary Microadenomas, pp 367-382. Academic Press, London, New York.

Lundin L, Liunghall S, Wide L & Bostrom J (1978): Bromocriptine therapy in eleven patients with acromegaly. Acta Endocrinol (Copenh), Suppl 216: 207-216.

Maneschi F (1980): Reappraisal of bromocriptine treatment for acromegaly. Horm Res 12: 191-205.

Maneschi F, Navalesi R, Pilo R & Paci A (1978): [^{125}I]-hGH metabolism in acromegaly: effects of chronic treatment with 2-Br-Alph-ergocryptine. J Clin Endocrinol Metab 47: 110-118.

Marek J, Sramkova J, Schullerova M, Stephan J & Schreiberova O (1981): Long-term treatment of acromegaly with lisuride: differences of the effect on growth hormone and somatomedin. Endokrinologie 2/3: 175-185.

Mellander S & Nordenfelt I (1976): Peripheral and central circulatory effects of dihydroergotamine. Postgrad Med J 52: Suppl 1: 17-20.

Moriondo P, Travaglini P, Rodena M, Beck-Peccoz P, Contin Puglisi F, Ambrosi B & Faglia G (1980): Prolactin secretion in acromegaly. In: Faglia G, Giovanelli MA & MacLeod RM (eds). Pituitary Microadenomas, pp 367-382. Academic Press, London, New York.

Nieuwenhuijzen Kruseman AC, Bots GThAM, Roelfsema F, Frölich M & van Dulken H (1983): Immunocytochemical growth hormone and prolactin in pituitary adenomas causing acromegaly and their relationship to basal serum hormone levels and the growth hormone response to thyrotrophin releasing hormone. Clin Endocrinol (Oxf) 19: 1-8.

Oppizzi G, Botalla L, Verde G, Cozzi R, Liuzzi A & Chiodini PG (1980): Homogeneity in the growth hormone-lowering effect of dopamine and somatostatin in acromegaly. J Clin Endocrinol Metab 51: 616-619.

Pelkonen R, Ylikahri R & Karonen SL (1980): Bromocriptine treatment of patients with acromegaly resistant to conventional therapy. Clin Endocrinol (Oxf) 12: 219-224.

Quabbe HJ (1982): Treatment of acromegaly by transsphenoidal operation, 90-Yttrium implantation and bromocriptine: results in 230 patients. Clin Endocrinol (Oxf) 16: 107-119.

Roelfsema F, Goslings BM, Frölich M, Moolenaar AJ, VanSeters AP & VanSlooten H (1979): The influence of bromocriptine on serum levels of growth hormone and other pituitary hormones and its metabolic effects in active acromegaly. Clin Endocrinol (Oxf) 11: 235-244.

Sachdev Y, Tunbridge WMG, Weightman DR, Gomez-Pan A, Duns A & Hall R (1975): Bromocriptine treatment in acromegaly. Lancet 2: 1164-1168.

Schwinn G, Dirks H, McIntosh C & Köbberling J (1977): Metabolic and clinical studies on patients with acromegaly treated with bromocriptine over 22 months. Eur J Clin Invest 7: 101-107.

Shalet SM, Price DA, Beardwell CG, Mindel A & MacFarlane IA (1980): Growth hormone and somatomedin levels in acromegalics treated with bromocriptine. Horm Res 12: 121-129.

Summers VK, Hipklin LJ, Diver MJ & Davis JC (1975): Treatment of acromegaly with bromocriptine. J Clin Endocrinol Metab 40: 904-906.

Thorner MO, Chait A, Aitken M, Benker G, Bloom SR, Mortimer CH, Sanders P, Stuart-Mason A & Besser GM (1975): Bromocriptine treatment of acromegaly. Br Med J 1: 299-303.

Wass JAH, Thorner MO, Morris DV, Rees LH, Stuart-Mason A, Jones AE & Besser GM (1977): Long-term treatment of acromegaly with bromocriptine. Br Med J 1: 875-878.

Wass JAH, Clemmons DR, Underwood LE, Barrow I, Besser GM & VanWyk JJ (1982): Changes in circulating somatomedin-C levels in bromocriptine-treated acromegaly. Clin Endocrinol (Oxf) 17: 369-377.

CHAPTER IV

Bromocriptine therapy in acromegaly: effects on plasma GH levels, somatomedin-C levels and clinical activity

J.W.R. Nortier, R.J.M. Croughs, J.H.H. Thijssen and F. Schwarz

SUMMARY

Thirty-one patients with active acromegaly were treated with 10-20 mg bromocriptine daily for a period of 6-9 months. The clinical response was evaluated both by a subjective "score of symptoms", and by a combined subjective and objective "clinical and metabolic improvement score" (c-m score). The biochemical response was evaluated both by measurement of the mean of 4 plasma growth hormone (GH) determinations during the day and by measurement of plasma somatomedin-C (Sm-C) concentration.

The clinical response as assessed by both methods showed a better correlation with changes in plasma GH levels (respectively $r = 0.33$; $r = 0.50$) than with changes in Sm-C levels ($r = 0.20$; $r = 0.36$). The study confirms that in some patients clinical improvement is not accompanied by a decrease of plasma GH concentrations. However, it is not possible to identify a subgroup of patients that shows a clinical improvement with a decrease of Sm-C levels, but whose plasma GH levels remain constant. It is concluded that measurement of plasma GH levels still appears to be the most useful biochemical assessment of disease activity in bromocriptine treated acromegaly.

INTRODUCTION

In the treatment of acromegaly therapeutic results are commonly assessed by the determination of plasma GH levels. Somatomedin activity determined by bio-assay and radio-receptor assay has been found to be elevated in some studies (Daughaday et al., 1959; Almqvist et al., 1961; Takano et al., 1976; Wiedemann et al., 1979) but to be normal in other studies (Holdaway et al., 1978; Shalet et al., 1980). Recently, a highly specific radioimmunoassay for somatomedin-C (Sm-C) has been developed (Furlanetto et al., 1977). As the growth promoting effects of GH are mediated by somatomedins, the question arises whether it would be appropriate to use the Sm-C radioimmunoassay instead of plasma GH determinations for the evaluation of acromegalic activity. Reports, correlating the results of both plasma GH levels and Sm-C levels with clinical activity, have been conflicting (Clemmons et al., 1979; Moses et al., 1981; Stonesifer et al., 1981; Wass et al., 1982).

The assay method for Sm-C used by the various investigators was virtually the same but their methods of clinical assessment varied. In one study clinical activity was assessed by heel-pad thickness and glucose tolerance (Clemmons et al. 1979) whereas in another study the response to bromocriptine therapy was assessed by a clinical and metabolic improvement score, which was obtained by adding points for subjective improvement of symptoms and objective improvement of ring size and glucose tolerance (Wass et al., 1982). In two other studies the clinical response to therapy was evaluated either by asking the patients to complete a questionnaire listing symptoms (Stonesifer et al., 1981) or by an assessment of clinical status by objective and subjective changes of disease activity on a 0-4$^+$ scale (Moses et al., 1981).

For practical purposes it is important to know whether Sm-C levels are superior to GH levels in the assessment of clinical activity and the response to treatment of acromegaly. We therefore compared Sm-C and plasma GH levels by applying two methods of clinical evaluation: one subjective, the other a combination of subjective and objective criteria of disease activity.

Furthermore, in some patients somatomedin A (Sm-A) was measured by a radioreceptor assay. Sm-A consists of a mixture of insuline like growth factor I (IGF-I) which is identical to Sm-C and insulin like growth factor II (IGF-II). The plasma concentrations of IGF-I/Sm-C are more GH dependent than those of IGF-II (Zapf et al., 1978; van Wyk et al., 1980; Daughaday, 1982).

PATIENTS AND METHODS

The study was carried out on 31 acromegalic patients. These patients all showed clinical activity with failure to suppress plasma GH levels to less than 4 mÛl after a 75 gram glucose load.

Sixteen had been treated with external irradiation, 7 with surgery, 4 with both surgery and external irradiation, 4 were yet untreated. Eleven patients had partial or complete pituitary insufficiency and all received appropriate hormonal replacement.

Bromocriptine was given in increasing doses up to a stage that the patients could tolerate four times daily 2.5 mg with their meals without showing side-effects.

This treatment was continued for a period of 6 months in those patients showing a decrease of the mean basal GH level of at least 50%. In the other patients it was tried to increase the dose to 20 mg daily after 3 months and to continue this treatment for a further period of 6 months (table 1).

Before and at the end of the treatment period of 6-9 months the clinical status was evaluated on the basis of two methods: by subjective improvement of acromegalic symptoms only and by a combination of subjective clinical improvement and objective improvement of glucose tolerance and ring size.

The improvement of symptoms only was recorded by comparing a clinical score of maximal 14 points before and at the end of the treatment period. This score was obtained by adding the scores for each symptom according to the degree of severity in the following way: acral swelling 0-3 points, hyperhidrosis 0-2 points, headache 0-2 points, weakness/fatigue 0-2 points, paraesthesia 0-1 point, joint/muscle pain 0-1 point, sleep-apnoe 0-1 points, sexual insufficiency 0-1 point, hirsutism/hypertrichosis 0-1 point.

The assessment of clinical improvement on the basis of subjective and objective criteria of disease activity was made in the same way as has been published by Wass et al. (1982) (table 2). Similar to their report clinical improvement was arbitrarily defined by a clinical and metabolic (c-m) score of 3 or greater. Finger circumference was measured with a set of jeweller's rings. Glucose tolerance was assessed by measuring blood glucose at 0, 30, 60, 90, 120 and 150 minutes after an oral glucose load of 75 gram.

Plasma GH levels were determined at 08.30 h (fasting), 13.00 h, 17.00 h and 19.00 h before bromocriptine treatment and after 6-9 months during continued bromocriptine administration but not simultaneously with the oral glucose tolerance tests. The mean value of these samples was used as the index of the GH secretion during the day. Before and at the end of the treatment period Sm-C was measured in all patients and Sm-A in 10 patients from plasma samples obtained at 08.30 h on the day of the GH day curve.

GH (1 μg/l = 2 mU/l MRC 66/217) was measured by radioimmunoassay as reported before (Nortier et al., 1984).

Blood glucose was measured with the hexokinase method using a Technicon Autoanalyzer II. All determinations were done in duplicate.

Plasma Sm-C was measured by radioimmunoassay by Endocrine Sciences, Tarzana, California, as described by Furlanetto et al. (1977). At Endocrine Sciences, specific somatomedin-C/IGF-I levels are measured in serum after chromatography on Sephadex G-50 columns in 0.25 M formic acid. This acid chromatography step yields a fraction containing over 95% of the applied Sm-C/IGF-I activity with no detectable binding protein activity (Kemp et al., 1981). Fractions containing Sm-C/IGF-I are then lyophilized prior to radioimmunoassay. Assay of acid chromatographed serum is performed using an antiserum developed in rabbits against the 12 amino acid C-peptide fragment of IGF-I (Hintz et al., 1980). This antiserum has no

Table 1. Patient data

Patient no.	Age yrs	Sex	Previous therapy[1]	Pituitary hormone deficiency	Basal GH[2] mU/l	Bromocriptine dose (mg)	Therapy duration (months)
Poor clinical response							
1. Bee	36	M	TFS, Irr, 1979	FSH, LH	43	20	9
2. Ros	48	M	TSS, 1971	ACTH, TSH, LH, FSH	72	20	9
3. Wie	31	F	TFS, Irr, 1977	ACTH, TSH, LH, FSH	6	20	9
4. Pel	35	M	TFS, 1966 TFS, Irr, 1969	ACTH, TSH, LH, FSH	40	20	9
5. Kip	65	M	Irr, 1977		30	10	6
6. Aup	57	F	TSS, 1970		14	10	9
Clinical improvement, reduction GH < 7%							
7. Bri	54	M	TSS, 1964		30	20	9
8. Lok	41	M	TSS, 1971	ACTH, LH, FSH	59	20	9
9. Lel	52	M	Irr, 1979		16	20	9
10. Age	71	F	Irr, 1954		7	20	9
11. Eek	35	M	Irr, 1976		6	20	9
12. Dijk	68	F			24	10	9
Clinical improvement, reduction GH 32 – 50%							
13. Zie	41	F	Irr, 1965		47	20	9
14. Jan	47	F	TFS, 1967	ACTH, LH, FSH	24	20	9
15. Jac	37	F	Irr, 1975		23	20	9
16. Swa	51	F	TFS, 1960 Irr, 1970	TSH	20	20	9
17. Mas	54	F	Irr, 1976		17	20	9
18. Goe	45	F	Irr, 1979		14	20	9
19. May	63	F			16	10	9
20. Tan	44	M	Irr, 1980	ACTH, TSH, LH, FSH	28	20	9

Clinical improvement, reduction GH > 53%							
21. Sleu	50	F	Irr, 1974		207	10	6
22. Vle	32	M	Irr, 1976		52	20	9
23. Ven	37	F	Irr, 1975		38	10	6
24. Nob	66	F	TSS, 1964	ACTH, TSH, LH, FSH	33	10	6
25. Kel	65	M	Irr, 1961		28	20	9
26. Beu	31	F	Irr, 1977		20	20	9
27. Vla	50	M	Irr, 1977	FSH, LH	15	10	6
28. Pal	41	F	Irr, 1978		11	20	9
29. Wij	74	F			48	10	6
30. Joo	58	M			13	20	9
31. Boo	65	M	TSS, 1965	ACTH, TSH, LH, FSH	71	10	6

[1] TSS, transsphenoidal surgery; TFS, transfrontal surgery; Irr, external irradiation.
[2] Mean of 4 determinations during the day.

Table 2. Clinical and metabolic score

Symptoms and signs	Score
Subjective	
Excessive sweating: abolished	2
Excessive sweating: reduced	1
Improvement in facial features	1
Reduction in foot size	1
Objective	
Reduction in ring circumference	
by 3 mm	3
by 1.5–3 mm	2
by 0.6–1.5 mm	1
Reduction in area under the glucose tolerance curve:	
by 40%	3
by 20–40%	2
by 5–20%	1
by 0– 5%	0
Increase in area	–1

detectable cross-reactivity with IGF-II. Purified preparations of IGF-I are used for both iodination and standards. The assay is performed under equilibrium conditions with an 18 hour incubation at 4°C. Separation of free and bound hormone is achieved using second antibody- polyethylene glycol. All acid chromatographed serum extracts are assayed in duplicate at three dilutions to insure linearity with the purified IGF-I standard. A normal adult serum pool served as the reference standard. This pool is comprised of the sera of 99 males and females ranging in age from 18-88 years and has been arbitrarily designated to contain 1.0 U/ml of somatomedin-C activity. For subjects aged 26-85 years (n = 38) the upper level of normal is 1.73 U/ml (1.05 + 2 SD).

Sm-A was measured by Kabivitrum laboratories (Stockholm, Sweden) with a placental radioreceptor- assay according to Takano et al. (1976). It is calibrated so that 1 U/ml approximates the mean concentration of normal adults.

RESULTS

Plasma levels of Sm-C before and during bromocriptine therapy were compared with mean plasma GH levels and with the patients' clinical responses assessed by the two methods of clinical evaluation. There was no significant correlation between Sm-C levels and mean plasma GH levels before bromocriptine therapy ($r = 0.25$), whereas during chronic bromocriptine therapy a weak but significant correlation was apparent ($r=0.44, p<0.05$, figure 1 A, B). When the percentage change of the mean plasma GH level during chronic bromocriptine therapy was correlated with the percentage change of Sm-C, about the same degree of correlation was found ($r = 0.45$, figure 1C).

There was no significant correlation between the percentage change of the score of symptoms with the percentage change of the mean plasma GH level ($r = 0.33$) or the percentage change of Sm-C ($r = 0.20$). The correlation between the percentage change of the mean plasma GH level and the clinical response was significant when this was evaluated by the c-m score ($r=0.50$, $p < 0.01$). There was a somewhat better correlation between the c-m score than between the score of symptoms and the percentage change of Sm-C ($r=0.36$ vs $r = 0.20$). However, the results obtained with the two methods of clinical evaluation were in rather good agreement ($r = 0.74$, $p < 0.001$, figure 2).

On the basis of the clinical assessment (c-m score) and the reduction of the mean plasma GH level the patients could be divided into four groups (table 3).

1. A group of six patients (no. 1-6) who had a poor clinical response (c-m score 0-2). When in these patients the score of symptoms was used as the method of clinical evaluation a poor clinical response was also found (decrease by 0-33%). In one of these patients (no. 5) GH levels decreased

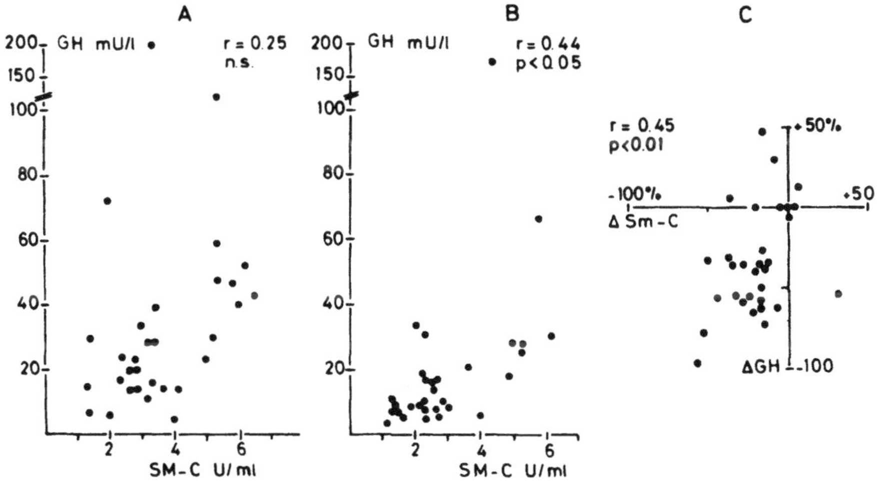

Fig. 1.

A,B. Correlation between the mean of 4 plasma GH determinations during the day (vertical axis) and Sm-C concentrations (horizontal axis) before (A) and during (B) chronic bromocriptine therapy.

C. Correlation between the percentage change of the mean plasma GH level during the day (vertical axis) and the percentage change of Sm-C (horizontal axis).

Table 3. Changes of mean plasma GH levels, somatomedin-C levels and of clinical response.

Patient no.	Mean plasma GH (mU/l)			Somatomedin C (U/ml)			Score of symptoms (range 0–14)			Clinical and metabolic (c-m) improvement score (range 0–10)
	B[1]	D[1]	Δ GH (%)	B[1]	D[2]	Δ Sm-C (%)	B[1]	D[2]	Δ score (%)	
Poor clinical response										
1. Bee	43	26	-40	6.5	5.2	-20	6	4	-33	2
2. Ros	122	179	+47	5.3	4.4	-17	6	5	-17	0
3. Wie	6	6	0	2.0	1.6	-20	8	8	0	2
4. Pel	40	29	-28	6	5	-17	6	6	0	1
5. Kip	30	11	-63	1.4	1.3	-7	3	3	0	2
6. Aup	14	9	-36	2.6	2.1	-19	9	7	-22	1
Clinical improvement, reduction GH < 7%										
7. Bri	30	28	-7	5.2	5.2	0	10	8	-20	4
8. Lok	59	67	+13	5.3	5.7	+7	9	6	-33	5
9. Lel	17	17	0	2.3	2.3	0	6	3	-50	6
10. Age	7	7	0	1.3	1.3	0	7	4	-43	4
11. Eek	6	6	0	4.0	4.0	0	8	3	-62	6
12. Dijk	24	31	+30	2.4	2.2	-8	9	6	-33	4
Clinical improvement, reduction GH 32 – 50%										
13. Zie	47	30	-36	5.9	6.1	+5	11	7	-36	5
14. Jan	24	16	-33	5.0	2.5	-50	6	3	-50	5
15. Jac	23	15	-35	2.8	2.5	-11	7	3	-57	4
16. Swa	20	10	-50	2.7	2.2	-18	8	5	-37	5
17. Mas	16	10	-37	3.3	2.9	-12	10	7	-33	3
18. Goe	14	9	-36	2.9	1.9	-35	5	3	-40	4
19. May	14	9	-36	4.1	3.0	-27	5	2	-60	5
20. Tan	28	19	-32	3.3	2.2	-33	10	10	0	3

Clinical improvememt, reduction GH > 53%										
21. Sle	207	9	-96	3.3	1.4	-58	10	3	-70	9
22. Vle	52	18	-65	6.2	4.9	-21	2	2	0	5
23. Ven	39	17	-56	3.4	2.6	-24	6	2	-67	7
24. Nob	34	8	-77	3.0	1.4	-54	9	4	-56	8
25. Kel	28	8	-61	3.2	2.6	-19	8	4	-50	7
26. Beu	20	8	-60	2.7	2.2	-19	10	4	-60	7
27. Vla	15	4	-73	1.3	1.1	-15	7	3	-57	4
28. Pal	11	5	-55	3.1	2.3	-26	8	4	-50	7
29. Wij	48	21	-56	5.4	3.6	-33	5	2	-60	9
30. Joo	14	6	-57	3.7	2.7	-27	7	3	-57	6
31. Boo	72	34	-53	2.0	2.5	+25	11	6	-45	4

[1] B, before bromocriptine treatment.

[2] D, during bromocriptine treatment.

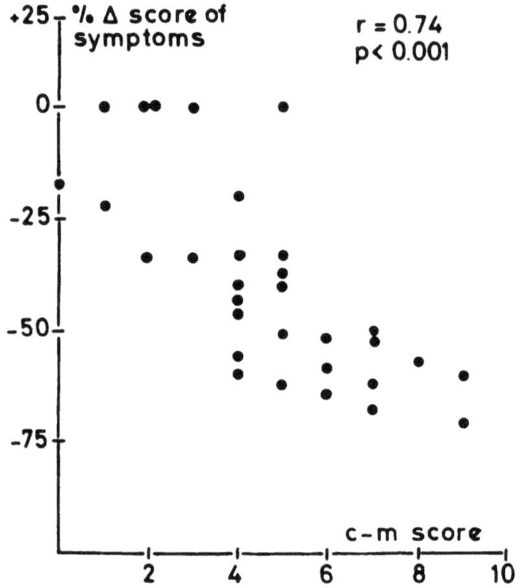

Fig. 2. Correlation between the percentage change of the score of symptoms (vertical axis) and the clinical and metabolic improvement score (horizontal axis) during chronic bromocriptine therapy.

by more than 50%, in three patients (no. 1, 4, 6) GH levels decreased by 25-50%, in one patient (no. 3) no change was noted and in one patient (no. 2) GH levels increased. Sm-C levels decreased by 7-20% during chronic bromocriptine treatment.

2. Six patients (no. 7-12) who had a clinical response to bromocriptine reflected by c-m score of 4-6 and a decrease of the score of symptoms of 20-62%, but whose plasma GH levels were practically unchanged or even increased somewhat. Sm-C levels were unchanged in 4 patients (no. 7, 9-11), while in 2 patients (no. 8, 12) only minor changes were observed.
3. Eight patients (no. 13-20) who responded to bromocriptine therapy clinically with a c-m score of 3-5 and with a decrease of the score of symptoms of 33-60% in 7 of them (no. 13-19). Plasma GH levels decreased by 32-50%. Sm-C levels decreased in 7 patients by 11-50% (no. 14-20); in one patient (no. 13) practically no change was found.
4. Eleven patients (no. 21-31) who had a clinical response to bromocriptine therapy with a c-m score of 4-9 and with a decrease of the score of symptoms of 45-70% in 10 patients (no. 21, 23-31) and with a decrease of the mean plasma GH level of more than 53%. Sm-C levels decreased by 15-58% in ten patients (no. 21-30); in one patient (no. 31) a 25% increase of Sm-C was measured.

Before bromocriptine therapy was instituted, the Sm-C levels were normal in 3 patients (no. 5, 10, 27) whereas mean plasma GH levels were at that time respectively 29, 7 and 15 mU/l. During bromocriptine therapy a decrease to normal from the previous – clearly elevated – Sm-C levels was only found in 2 patients (no. 21, 24). These two patients also showed an excellent GH and clinical response.

The results of the Sm-A measurements are listed in table 4 together with the Sm-C values. Good correlations were present between Sm-C and Sm-A values before and at the end of the treatment period ($r = 0.71$, $p < 0.05$; $r = 0.97$, $p < 0.001$) and also between the change of Sm-C and Sm-A during chronic bromocriptine treatment ($r = 0.74$, $p < 0.05$). The results support the reliability of the Sm-C values used in our study.

DISCUSSION

In the present study the clinical response to chronic bromocriptine therapy in 31 acromegalic patients was assessed both by a subjective "score of symptoms" and by the combined subjective "clinical and metabolic improvement score" (c-m score). It seems appropriate to include objective criteria of disease activity when a clinical assessment of acromegaly is made. The correlation between the results obtained with the two methods of clinical evaluation was good ($r = 0.74$, $p < 0.001$).

The biochemical response to chronic bromocriptine treatment was assessed by averaging four plasma GH determinations during the day and by the

Table 4.

Patient no.	Sm-A B[1]	Sm-A D[2]	Δ SmA (%)	SmC B[1]	Sm-C D[2]	Δ Sm-C (%)
5. Kip	1.3	1.1	-15	1.4	1.3	-7
13. Zie	4.0	3.4	-15	5.9	6.1	+5
14. Jan	3.7	2.0	-46	5.0	2.5	-50
19. May	4.0	2.2	-45	4.1	3.0	-27
20. Tan	1.8	1.3	-28	3.3	2.2	-33
22. Vle	3.1	2.8	-10	6.2	4.9	-21
24. Nob	3.9	1.1	-72	3.0	1.4	-54
27. Vla	1.1	1.2	+9	1.3	1.1	-15
29. Wij	6.3	2.0	-68	5.4	3.6	-33
30. Joo	3.0	2.0	-33	3.7	2.7	-27
Mean change ± SEM			-32 ± 8			-26 ± 6

[1] B, before bromocriptine treatment.
[2] D, during bromocriptine treatment.

measurement of Sm-C. In general, plasma GH levels in acromegalics show much less circadian variation than in normal subjects. It is therefore justified to average four values obtained during the day and to use the mean as an index of GH secretion. Sm-C has a half-life of 20 hours. Therefore, one determination per day must be sufficient.

Changes of the mean plasma GH-levels correlated better than changes of Sm-C levels with the clinical response as assessed by the two different methods.

It was not possible to confirm the findings of Wass et al. (1982) who could identify a subgroup of patients showing clinical improvement with a decrease of Sm-C levels but without reduction in GH values. In our population 6 patients (no. 7-12) showed clinical improvement without hardly any reduction in the GH secretion, but Sm-C levels also remained unchanged. Our findings are more in agreement with the study of Moses et al. (1981) who reported good clinical responses to chronic bromocriptine therapy in 6 of 7 acromegalic patients with considerable decreases of GH levels and only small decreases of Sm-C levels in 5 of them. In another study by Stonesifer et al. (1981) there were more discrepancies between clinical activity and Sm-C than between clinical activity and GH determinations.

Although Sm-C levels might show less fluctuation than plasma GH levels, it would seem "a priori" that a direct tumour product would be a better marker of tumour activity than a substance produced under the influence of that tumour product in the peripheral tissues. Thus caution should be exercised if Sm-C levels are utilized to assess disease activity in acromegalic patients (Daughaday, 1979).

In the present study measurement of Sm-C is not superior to the mean of 4 plasma GH levels, measured at fixed intervals during the day, in evaluating the clinical response to chronic bromocriptine therapy. It is concluded that GH determinations remain the best biochemical parameters of disease activity in bromocriptine treated acromegaly.

REFERENCES

Almqvist, S., Ikkos, D. & Luft, R. (1961) Studies on sulfation factor (SF) activity of human serum: serum SF in hypopituitarism and acromegaly. Acta Endocrinologica, 36, 577-595.

Clemmons, D.R., Van Wyk, J.J., Ridgway, E.C., Kliman, B., Kjellberg, R.N. & Underwood, L.E. (1979) Evaluation of acromegaly by radioimmunoassay of somatomedin-C. New England Journal of Medicine, 301, 1138-1142.

Daughaday, W.H., Salman, W.D. & Alexander, F. (1959) Sulfation factor activity of sera from patients with pituitary disorders. Journal of Clinical Endocrinology and Metabolism 19, 743-758.

Daughaday, W.H. (1979) New criteria for evaluation of acromegaly. New England Journal of Medicine 301, 1175.

Daughaday, W.H. (1982) Divergence of binding sites, in vitro action and secretory regulation of the somatomedin peptides, IGF-I and IGF-II (41.428). Proceedings of the Society for Experimental Biology and Medicine 170, 257-263.

Furlanetto, R.W., Underwood, L.E., Van Wyk, J.J. & d'Ercole, A.J. (1977) Estimation of somatomedin C levels in normals and patients with pituitary disease by radioimmunoassay. Journal of Clinical Investigation 60, 648-657.

Hintz, R.L., Liu, F., Marshall, L.B. & Chang, D. (1980) Interaction of somatomedin C with an antibody directed against the C-peptide region of insulin-like growth factor I. Journal of Clinical Endocrinology and Metabolism 50, 405-407.

Holdaway, J.M., Frengky, P.A., Scott, D.J. & Ibbertson, J.K. (1978) Bromocriptine treatment of acromegaly persisting following conventional therapy. Clinical Endocrinology 8, 45-54.

Moses, A.C., Molitsch, M.E., Sawin, C.T., Jackson, I.M.D., Biller, B.J., Furlanetto, R. & Reichlin, S. (1981) Bromocriptine therapy in acromegaly: use in patients resistant to conventional therapy and effect on serum levels of somatomedin-C. Journal of Clinical Endocrinology and Metabolism 53, 752-758.

Nortier, J.W.R., Croughs, R.J.M., Thijssen, J.H.H. & Schwarz, F. (1984) Plasma growth hormone suppressive effect of bromocriptine in acromegaly. Evaluation by plasma GH day profiles and plasma GH concentrations during oral glucose tolerance tests. Clinical Endocrinology 20, 565-571.

Shalet, S.M., Price, D.A., Beardwell, C.G., Mindel, A. & MacFarlane, J.A. (1980) Growth hormone and somatomedin levels in acromegalics treated with bromocriptine. Hormone Research 12, 121-129.

Stonesifer, L.D., Jordan, R.M. & Kohler, P.O. (1981) Somatomedin-C in treated acromegaly: poor correlation with growth hormone and clinical response. Journal of Clinical Endocrinology and Metabolism 53, 931-934.

Takano, K., Hall, K., Ritzen, M., Ischius, L. & Sievertsson, H. (1976) Somatomedin-A in human serum determined by radioreceptor assay. Acta Endocrinologica 82, 449-459.

Van Wyk, J.J., Svoboda, M.E., Underwood, L.E. (1980) Evidence from radio-ligand assays that somatomedin-C and insulin-like growth factor I are similar to each other and different from other somatomedins. Journal of Clinical Endocrinology and Metabolism 50, 206-208.

Wass, J.A.H., Clemmons, D.R., Underwood, L.E., Barrow, J., Besser, G.M. & Van Wyk, J.J. (1982) Changes in circulating somatomedin-C levels in bromocriptine- treated acromegaly. Clinical Endocrinology 17, 369-377.

Wiedemann, E., Uthne, K., Tang, R.G., Spencer, M., Saito, T. & Linfoot, J.A. (1979) Serum somatomedin activity by rat cartilage bio-assay and human placental membrane radioreceptor assay in acromegaly and Cushing's disease. In: Somatomedins and Growth (eds. G. Giordano, J.J. Van Wyk & F. Minuto) pp 289-294. Academic Press, New York.

Zapf, J., Rinderknecht, E., Humbol, R.E. & Froesch, E.R. (1978) Non-suppressible insulin-like activity (NSILA) from human serum: recent accomplishments and their physiological implications. Metabolism 50, 206-108.

CHAPTER V

Gel filtration studies of plasma growth hormone in bromocriptine treated acromegaly: correlations with somatomedin-C and clinical response

J.W.R. Nortier, R.J.M. Croughs, G.H. Donker, J.H.H. Thijssen and F. Schwarz

SUMMARY

Eleven patients with active acromegaly were treated with 10-20 mg bromocriptine daily for a period of 6-9 months. The clinical response was evaluated by a "clinical and metabolic improvement score". The biochemical response was evaluated by measurement of both the mean plasma growth hormone (GH) level during the day and the somatomedin-C (Sm-C) concentration.

Before and at the end of the treatment period plasma samples were fractionated by Sephadex G-100 chromatography in order to study the effects of chronic bromocriptine treatment on the concentrations of total immunoreactive GH and its different molecular forms.

The main observations may be summarized as follows:

1. Three immunoreactive components are observed on Sephadex chromatography, corresponding to molecular weight above 100.000 (big big GH), 40.000-60.000 (big GH) and 20.000-22.000 (little GH).
2. Bromocriptine treatment preferentially induces a reduction of little GH. There is a very good correlation between the decrease of little GH and total GH and both provide a significant correlation with the clinical response.
3. The correlation between the decrease of Sm-C values and the decrease of little and total GH as well as the correlation between the decrease of Sm-C and the clinical response is poor.

It is concluded that a) measurement of little GH is not superior to the determination of total GH in the assessment of disease activity of bromocriptine treated acromegalic patients; b) both methods are superior to the measurement of plasma Sm-C levels; c) a clinical response which is out of proportion to the fall of total GH and which can be explained by a preferential reduction of little GH, has not been observed in our investigations.

INTRODUCTION

It is well established that plasma GH levels do not always correlate with the clinical activity of acromegaly (Kanis et al., 1974; Mims et al., 1974). It has been suggested that somatomedin-C (Sm-C) concentrations correlate better with clinical status than does plasma GH (Clemmons et al., 1979; Wass et al., 1982), although this has not been found by others (Moses et al., 1981; Stonesifer et al., 1981) and could also not be confirmed by our group (chapter IV).

The biologically most active monomeric form of GH (little GH) has a higher radioreceptor activity than larger molecular forms and in acromegalics this difference is even greater than in normal subjects (Gorden et al., 1976). It could therefore be expected that little GH would correlate better with clinical status and perhaps also with Sm-C than total GH.

Chronic treatment with the dopamine agonist bromocriptine has led to a distinct clinical improvement and a reduction of plasma GH levels in the majority of patients with active acromegaly (Sachdev et al., 1975; Thorner et al., 1975; Belforte et al., 1977; Wass et al., 1977; Schwinn et al., 1977; Pelkonen et al., 1980; Sachdev et al., 1981; Wass et al., 1982; Nortier et al., 1984). A preferential decrease of little GH has been reported during chronic bromocriptine therapy (Besser et al., 1976; Benker et al., 1979). In one study evidence was found for an increase of the clearance of monomeric GH by bromocriptine (Maneschi et al., 1978).

In this paper we present the results of an investigation in bromocriptine treated acromegalic patients into the relation between changes of the various molecular form of GH in relation to changes of Sm-C and to the clinical response.

PATIENTS AND METHODS

Eleven patients, 5 females and 6 males with active acromegaly, aged 32-74 years (mean 49 years) were studied. One patient was yet untreated, four had been treated with external irradiation, five with pituitary surgery and one with both surgery and external irradiation. Five patients had partial or complete pituitary insufficiency despite persistent acromegaly; all of them received appropriate hormonal replacement. They all showed clinical active acromegaly with glucose non-suppressible GH-levels. They were selected from a larger group of patients (chapter IV) on the basis of a mean plasma GH level during the day of more than 30 mU/l.

Before and during continued bromocriptine therapy, which had been given for 6-9 months, the following investigations were carried out:

a. Clinical status was evaluated by a clinical and metabolic (c-m) improvement score as described by Wass et al. (1982). This score was obtained by adding points for subjective improvements of symptoms (reduction in sweating, reduction in foot size and improvement in facial features) and objective improvements of ring size and glucose tolerance (range 0-10 points).

b. Plasma GH levels were determined at 08.30 h (fasting), 13.00 h, 17.00 h and 19.00 h. The mean values of these samples were used as the index of the GH secretion during the day.

c. Plasma Sm-C levels were measured at 08.30 h on the day of the GH day curve.

d. Sephadex G-100 chromatography of plasma GH. This investigation was carried out on plasma samples obtained at 08.30 h before bromocriptine treatment and 4 h after the morning dose of bromocriptine at the end of the treatment period. The latter timing was chosen in order to have a maximal effect of bromocriptine at the moment of sampling for fractionation.

Plasma GH (1 µg/l = 2 mU/l) was determined by radioimmunoassay as reported before (Nortier et al., 1984). The lower limit of detection was approximately 0.5 mU/l. Intra- and inter-assay variations were 6 and 7.9% (n = 31) respectively. The samples from each patient were measured in the same assay. All values have been expressed in units of the 1st IRP-HGH.

Somatomedin-C levels were measured by radioimmunoassay by Endocrine Sciences, Tarzana, California (Furlanetto et al., 1977). For subjects aged 26-85 years (n = 38) the upper level of normal is 1.73 U/ml (1.05 + 2 SD).

Fractionations were carried out at 4°C on a Sephadex G-100 column 85 × 1.5 cm, at a flow rate of 8.6 ml/h using a peristaltic pump and an automatic fraction collector.

A 0.01 M phosphate, 0.15 M sodium chloride buffer, pH 7.5, containing 0.1% bovine serum albumin and 0.02% sodiumazide was used for elution. The column was calibrated using blue dextran as a marker for the void volume (V_o 72 ml), albumin (MW 67.000, 85.5 ml, K_{av} 0.13), ovalbumin (MW 43.000, 95 ml, K_{av} 0.22), ^{125}I-GH (MW 21.500, 116 ml, K_{av} 0.41), ribonuclease (MW 13.700, 125 ml, K_{av} 0.52) and Na^{125}I as a marker for the salt peak (V_t 175 ml). K_{av} was calculated according to Laurent and Killander (1964) by the equation

$$K_{av} = \frac{V_e - V_o}{V_t - V_o}$$

where Ve represents the elution volume, Vt the total volume of the column and Vo the void volume. The volume applied to the column was 1 ml and consisted of 0.9 ml plasma and 0.1 ml purified ^{125}I-GH. To test the reproducibility of the procedure 1 ml plasma of a normal subject containing 112 mU/l

GH obtained after infusion with arginine was fractionated two times on separate days.

The sign-test for paired differences was used to compare results.

RESULTS

Recovery of immunoreactive GH ranged from 62-120% (table 1). Before and during chronic bromocriptine therapy 3 GH components were usually found with K_{av} values of 0.41 ± 0.01, 0.22 ± 0.03 and 0.06 ± 0.03 respresenting respectively little GH (MW 20.000-22.000), big GH (MW 40.000-60.000) and big big GH (MW > 100.000).

As is shown in table 1 before treatment with bromocriptine, little GH accounted for 40-76% (median 62%), big GH for 10-22% (median 15%) and big big GH for 0-37% (median 8%) of total immunoreactivity. Some immu-

Table 1. Recoveries of total GH after Sephadex *f*-100 chromatography and the distribution of the 3 molecular forms of GH.

Patient		Total GH mU/l	Recovery %	GH components, % of total GH		
				'big big'	'big'	'little'
1. Sie	B	236	110	5	18	75
	D	39	78	3	26	34
2. Wij	B	45	104	37	16	44
	D	12	108	33	16	41
3. Nob	B	27	111	4	19	53
	D	7	120	10	25	54
4. Boo	B	73	75	10	12	63
	D	31	81	12	15	54
5. Ven	B	27	74	8	22	59
	D	11	92	3	21	38
6. Vle	B	43	87	3	15	69
	D	34	115	11	29	49
7. Zie	B	48	66		12	66
	D	26	68	15	15	42
8. Bri	B	29	86	10	14	71
	D	26	62	6	8	68
9. Pel	B	40	78		10	40
	D	29	83	5	14	37
10. Lok	B	64	109	18	18	61
	D	70	105	18	12	64
11. Ros	B	132	111	11	10	76
	D	183	93	11	15	70

B, before bromocriptine treatment.
D, during bromocriptine treatment.

noreactivity was also detected in the elution volumes after little GH. These fractions showed no definite peaks, absolute values were only occasionally above 1 mU/l and no differences were found before or during chronic bromocriptine therapy. When these samples were assayed either as single fractions or pooled after lyophilization there was no parallelism with standard GH. In contrast, dilution curves of peak fractions of big big, big and little GH gave parallel response curves in the GH radioimmunoassay. In pure buffer solution, also after lyophilization no GH immunoreactivity could be demonstrated.

The reproducibility of the fractionations and assay procedures is illustrated by the results obtained from 2 fractionations on separate occasions on plasma samples of a normal subject (figure 1). The fractionation pattern obtained with plasma of 2 patients (no. 1 and 4) is shown in figures 2 and 3. Patient no. 1 shows a nearly complete disappearance of all GH components. In patient no. 4 there is a preferential decrease of little GH.

Mean plasma GH levels, Sm-C values, absolute concentrations of total, big big, big and little GH before and during chronic bromocriptine therapy are listed in table 2 together with the clinical response expressed by the c-m score. The mean decrease of little GH is 46%, that of big GH 6%. This difference is statistically significant. The mean decrease of big big GH was 9% with a very wide scatter. The correlation between the decrease of little

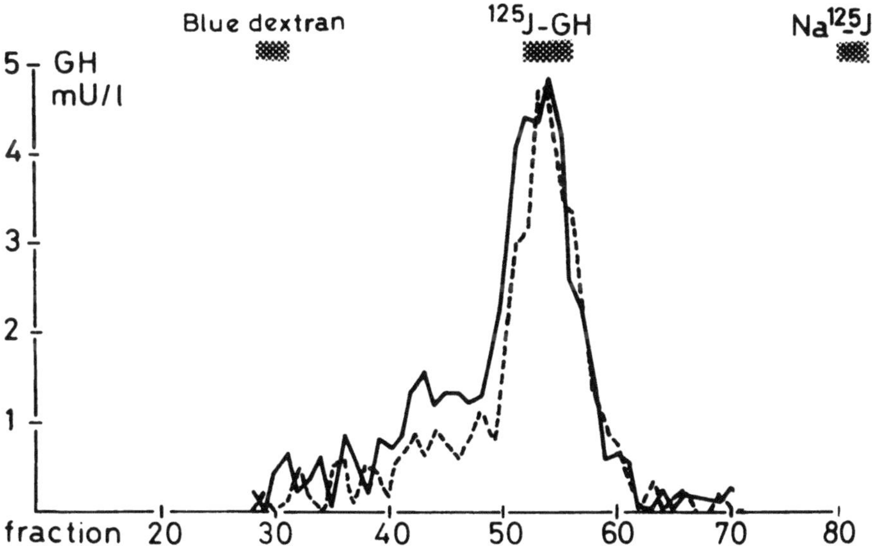

Fig. 1. Sephadex G-100 fractionation on two different occasions of a plasma sample obtained from a normal subject after arginine infusion.

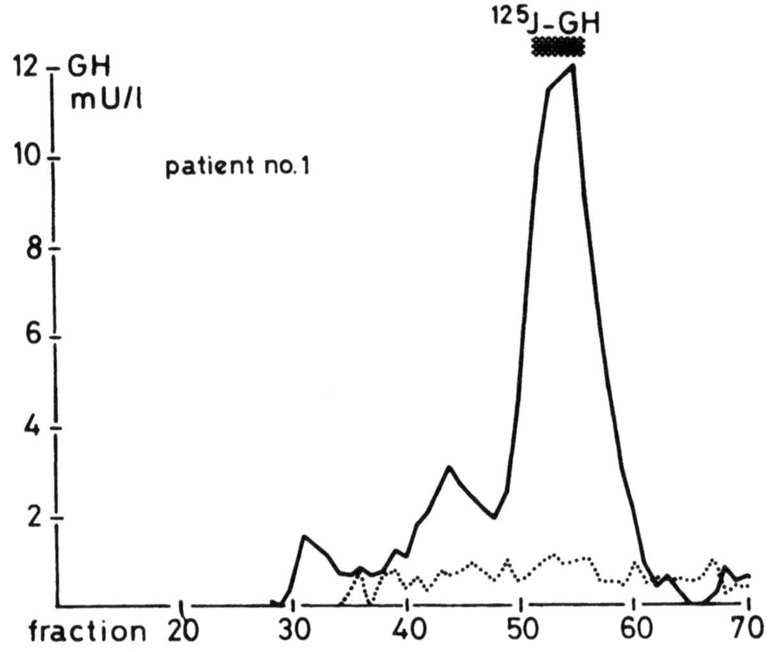

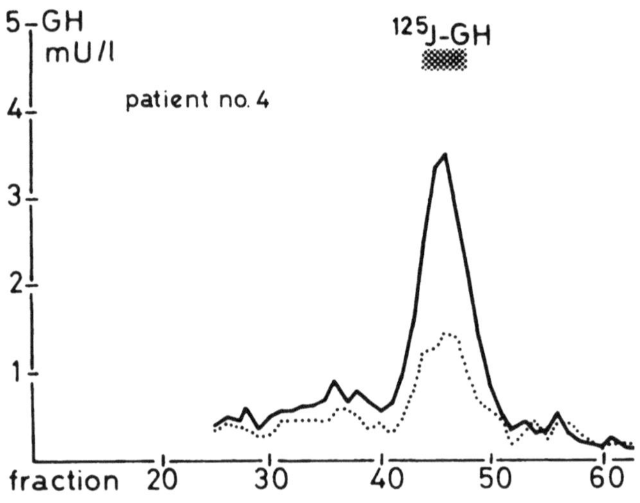

Figs. 2 Sephadex G-100 fractionations of patients no. 1 and 4 before (———) and during (- - -) chronic bromocriptine treatment.

Table 2. Percentage changes of the mean GH levels, somatomedin-C concentrations, the various molecular forms of GH and the clinical response.

Patient		Mean GH[1] mU/l	Sm-C U/l	GH components mU/l after Sephadex G 100 chromatography				c-m[2] score
				'big big'	'big'	'little'	'total'	
1. Sle	B	207	3.3	13	47	195	260	
	D	9	1.4	1	8	10	30	9
change	%	-96	-58	-92	-85	-95	-89	
2. Wij	B	48	5.4	17	7	21	47	
	D	21	3.6	4	2	5	13	9
change	%	-56	-33	-77	-71	-76	-72	
1. Nob	B	34	3.0	1	6	16	30	
	D	8	1.4	0	2	5	11	8
change	%	-77	-54	-100	-66	-69	-63	
4. Boo	B	72	2.0	5.5	7	35	55	
	D	34	2.5	3	4	13.5	25	4
change	%	-53	+25	-45	-43	-61	-65	
5. Ven	B	39	3.4	1	6	12	20	
	D	17	2.6	0	2	4	10	7
change	%	-56	-24	-100	-67	-67	-50	
6. Vle	B	52	6.2	1	5.5	25	37	
	D	18	4.9	4	11	19	39	5
change	%	-65	-21	+300	+100	-24	+5	
7. Zie	B	47	5.9	2	4	21	32	
	D	30	6.1	3	3	8	18	5
change	%	-36	+5	+50	-25	-67	-44	
8. Bri	B	30	5.2	2.5	3.5	18	25	
	D	28	5.2	1.0	2	11	16	4
change	%	-7	0	-60	-43	-39	-36	
9. Pel	B	40	6		1	12	31	
	D	29	5		3	9	24	1
change	%	-28	-17		+200	-25	-23	
10. Lok	B	59	5.3	13	13	43	70	
	D	67	5.7	13	9	47	73	5
change	%	+13	+7	0	-31	+9	+4	
11. Ros	B	122	5.3	16	15	111	146	
	D	179	4.4	19	25	119	170	0
change	%	+47	-17	+19	+67	+7	+16	
Mean		-38	-17	-9	-6**	-46*	-38	
change	%	±	±	±	±	±	±	
± SEM		13	8	35	27	10	10	

[1] Mean of 4 GH determinations during the day.

[2] c-m, clinical and metabolic improvement score (range 0-10 points).

B, before bromocriptine treatment.

D, during bromocriptine treatment.

* vs ** $p < 0.05$ (sign test).

GH and that of total GH was very good ($r = 0.94$, $p < 0.001$), that of either little GH or total GH with the change in Sm-C was poor ($r = 0.45$ and $r = 0.43$). Changes in little as well as in total GH showed about the same correlation with the clinical response expressed by the c-m score (respectively $r = 0.75$, $p < 0.01$ and $r = 0.72$, $p < 0.05$). The correlation of changes in Sm-C with the clinical response was only $r = 0.55$.

DISCUSSION

This study confirms the heterogeneity of plasma GH in acromegalic patients. The percentage of little GH (40-76%), big GH (10-22%) and big big GH (0-37%) are in agreement with those found by Benker et al. (1979). Goodman et al. (1972) and Gorden et al. (1976) found somewhat higher percentages for little GH (65-84% and 77-95%).

In addition, we found some immunoreactivity in elution volumes corresponding to molecular sizes smaller than little GH. It is questionable whether these fractions represent fragments which have retained some immunoreactivity or whether they are artefacts. Similar findings have only been reported in one previous study (Bala et al. 1970) in which extracts from large volumes of plasma were fractionated.

Since, particularly in acromegalic patients, little GH is known to have a higher radioreceptor activity than larger molecular forms of GH (Gorden et al., 1976), it has been suggested that the somatomedins, particularly Sm-C, correlate better with little GH than with total GH (Moses et al., 1981; Wass et al., 1982) and that the same holds for the clinical activity of acromegaly.

Our results do not support this supposition. Change of little GH did not correlate better with change of Sm-C than that of total GH. The correlation with clinical response was about the same whether little or total GH was used.

The situation that a decrease in little GH is partially or completely compensated by an increase in big big or big GH as has been described by Benker et al. (1979) appears to be an exception in the group of patients that was investigated in this study. It has been observed in some patients that the degree of clinical improvement is greater than would be expected from the apparent reduction in circulating GH (Sachdev et al., 1975; Belforte et al., 1977; Wass et al. 1977, 1982). This discrepancy has been explained in various ways. The most important mechanisms advanced are a selective reduction of Sm-C with unchanged GH secretion and alternatively a preferential reduction of little GH. Two of the 11 patients we investigated showed clinical improvement without a reduction of the mean plasma GH level (patient no. 8 and 10, table 2). In these patients Sm-C levels did not decrease and no selective reduction of little GH was found.

The present study confirms that little GH is preferentially suppressed during chronic bromocriptine therapy. But in none of our cases this mechanism could explain clinical improvement without a decrease in total plasma GH.

REFERENCES

Bala RM, Ferguson KA & Beck JC (1970): Plasma biological and immunoreactive human growth hormone-like activity. Endocrinology 87: 506-516.

Belforte L, Camanni F, Chiodini PG, Liuzzi A, Massara F, Molinatti GM, Müller EE, Silvestrini F (1977): Long-term treatment with 2 Br-alpha-ergocryptine in acromegaly. Acta Endocrinol (Copenh) 85: 235-248.

Benker G, Sandmann K, Tharandt L, Hackenberg K, Reinwein D (1979): Gel filtration studies of serum growth hormone in acromegaly following bromocriptine administration. Horm Res 11: 151-160.

Besser GM, Thorner MO, Wass JAH, Jones AE, Lowry P, Rees LH, Jones A (1976): Bromocriptine treatment of acromegaly. Q L Med 45: 695-696.

Clemmons DR, Van Wyk JJ, Ridgway EC, Kliman B, Kjellberg RN, Underwood LE (1979): Evaluation of acromegaly by radioimmunoassay of somatomedin-C. N Engl J Med 301: 1138-1142.

Furlanetto RW, Underwood LE, Van Wyk JJ, D'Ercole AJ (1977): Estimation of somatomedin-C levels in normals and patients with pituitary disease by radioimmunoassay. J Clin Invest 60: 648-657.

Gorden P, Lesniak MA, Eastman R, Hendricks C, Roth J (1976): Evidence for higher proportion of "little" growth hormone with increased radioreceptor activity in acromegalic plasma. J Clin Endocrinol Metab 43: 364-373.

Goodman AD, Tanenbaum R, Rabinowitz D (1972): Existence of two forms of immunoreactive growth hormone in human plasma. J Clin Endocrinol Metab 35: 868-878.

Kanis JA, Gillingham FJ, Harris P, Horn DB, Hunter WM, Redpath AT, Strong JA (1974): Clinical and laboratory study of acromegaly: assessment before and one year after treatment. Q J Med 43: 409-431.

Laurent TC, Killander J (1964): A theory of gel filtration and its experimental verification. J Chromat 14: 317-330.

Maneschi F, Mavalesi R, Pilo A, Paci A (1978): [^{125}I] hGH metabolism in acromegaly: effects of chronic treatment with 2-Br-Ergocriptine. J Clin Endocrinol Metab 47: 110-118.

Mims RB, Bethuna JE (1974): Acromegaly with normal fasting growth hormone concentrations but abnormal growth hormone regulation. Ann Intern Med 81: 781-784.

Moses AC, Molitch ME, Sawin CT, Jackson IMD, Biller BJ, Furlanetto R, Reichlin S (1981): Bromocriptine therapy in acromegaly: use in patients resistant to conventional therapy and effect on serum levels of somatomedin-C. J Clin Endocrinol Metab 53: 752-758.

Nortier JWR, Croughs RJM, Thijssen JHH & Schwarz F (1984): Plasma growth hormone suppressive effect of bromocriptine in acromegaly. Evaluation by plasma GH day profiles and plasma GH concentrations during oral glucose tolerance tests. Clin Endocrinol (Oxf) 20: 565-571.

Pelkonen R, Ylikahri R, Karonen SL (1980): Bromocriptine treatment of patients with acromegaly resistant to conventional therapy. Clin Endocrinol (Oxf) 12: 219-224.

Sachdev Y, Tunbridge WMG, Weightman DR, Gomez-Pan A, Duns A, Hall R (1975): Bromocriptine treatment in acromegaly. Lancet 2: 1164-1168.

Sachdev Y, Gopal K & Garg XK (1981): Bromocriptine therapy in acromegaly. A long-term review of 35 cases. Postgrad Med J 57: 210-216.

Schwinn G, Dirks H, McIntosh C, Köbberling J (1977): Metabolic and clinical studies on patients with acromegaly treated with bromocriptine over 22 months. Eur J Clin Invest 7: 101-107.

Stonesifer LD, Jordan RM, Kohler PO (1981): Somatomedin-C in treated acromegaly: Poor correlation with growth hormone and clinical response. J. Clin Endocrinol Metab 53: 931-934.

Thorner MO, Chait A, Aitken M, Benker G, Bloom SR, Mortimer CH, Sanders P, Stuart-Mason A, Besser GM (1975): Bromocriptine treatment of acromegaly. Br Med J 1: 299-303.

Wass JAH, Thorner MO, Morris DV, Rees LH, Stuart-Mason A, Jones AE, Besser GM (1977): Long-term treatment of acromegaly with bromocriptine. Br Med J 1: 875-878.

Wass JAH, Clemmons DR, Underwood LE, Barrow I, Besser GM, Van Wyk JJ (1982): Changes in circulating somatomedin-C levels in bromocriptine treated acromegaly. Clin Endocrinol (Oxf) 17: 369-377.

CHAPTER VI

No acute effect of pimozide on the plasma GH levels in acromegaly

J.W.R. Nortier, R.J.M. Croughs, G.H. Donker, J.H.H. Thijssen and F. Schwarz

Department of Endocrinology, State University of Utrecht, Catharijnesingel 101, Utrecht, The Netherlands

ABSTRACT

In 34 acromegalic patients either untreated or inadequately treated by surgery and/or radiotherapy the plasma GH levels and plasma Prl levels were determined during 8 h after the acute administration of the dopamine agonist bromocriptine and during 150 min after the administration of the dopamine antagonist pimozide.

A 50% or more suppression of the basal GH levels was arbitrarily defined as a positive response. Seventeen patients displayed a positive response to bromocriptine, 17 patients displayed a negative response to bromocriptine. Plasma Prl levels were elevated in 6 of 17 bromocriptine responders and in 2 of 17 bromocriptine non-responders. There was no difference in the plasma GH response to pimozide administration in the patients with a positive or a negative GH response to bromocriptine.

With one exception there was in no patient a positive GH response to pimozide. In further experiments the plasma GH response to pimozide was measured during 11 h in 6 bromocriptine sensitive and 6 bromocriptine insensitive patients. Again no difference was found between bromocriptine responders and non-responders. There was also no difference in the Prl response to bromocriptine or pimozide between GH responders and GH non-responders. The Prl response to pimozide was blunted in comparison to a control group.

The present study does not lend support to the idea that there is a fundamental difference in the degree of hypothalamic dopaminergic control

Acta Endocrinologica 1983, 103: 461–468

of GH or Prl secretion between bromocriptine sensitive and bromocriptine insensitive patients with acromegaly.

INTRODUCTION

The treatment of acromegaly by surgery or radiotherapy is often unsatisfactory. Plasma GH-levels frequently remain elevated and adjunctive therapy with the dopamine agonist bromocriptine results in clinical and biochemical amelioration in 50-80% of patients (Thorner et al. 1975; Sachdev et al. 1975; Belforte et al. 1977; Wass et al. 1977, 1982; Roelfsema et al. 1979; Pelkonen et al. 1980).

Thus, at least 20% of patients do not improve on bromocriptine treatment. It is thought that in this group of patients in whom dopamine agonists fail, hypothalamic control of GH secretion could still be operating and that the GH levels could then be reduced by anti-dopaminergic agents such as pimozide (Carmina et al. 1979).

The possibility that dopamine antagonists act directly at the pituitary level as was shown for the dopamine agonist bromocriptine in an in vitro study (Ishibashi & Yamaji 1978) should also be considered.

The aim of this study was to test this hypothesis by measuring the GH response to the administration of a single dose of pimozide in a large number of acromegalic patients either untreated or with persistent clinical and biochemical activity despite previous treatment in the same way as has been described by Carmina et al. (1979).

Furthermore, in a smaller group of patients the GH response to the administration of a single dose of pimozide was studied during a longer period than in the study by Carmina et al. (1979). The patients were divided in bromocriptine responders and non-responders according to the reduction of the GH level of more or less than 50% of the initial value after the administration of a single dose of bromocriptine (Liuzzi et al. 1974; Belforte et al. 1977).

As the prolactin secretion follows most closely the central dopaminergic tone, the response to pimozide of this hormone was measured in all patients tested in the same way as in the study by Carmina et al. (1979) and in half of the patients tested during a longer period.

PATIENTS AND METHODS

The study was carried out on 34 acromegalic patients. They all showed clinical activity with glucose non-suppressible GH levels. Seventeen had been treated with external irradiation, 8 with surgery, 3 with both surgery and external irradiation, 6 had not received any treatment at the time of the present study. Eleven patients had partial or complete pituitary insufficiency, all received appropriate hormonal replacement (Table 1).

Table 1. Patient data

Patient no.	Age yrs	Sex	Previous therapy[1]	Pituitary hormone deficiency	Basal GH[2] mU/l	Basal Prl[3] U/l
1. Kel	65	M	Irr, 1961		28	0.84
2. Nob	66	F	TSS, 1964	ACTH, TSH, LH, FSH	33	0.45
3. Boo	65	M	TSS, 1965	ACTH, TSH, LH, FSH	72	0.74
4. Ven	37	F	Irr, 1975		38	1.8
5. Vle	32	M	Irr, 1976		53	0.46
6. Bee	36	M	TFS, 1969 Irr, 1979	FSH, LH	43	2.25
7. Cet	40	F	TFS, 1979	TSH, ACTH	8	0.21
8. Aup	57	F	TSS, 1970		14	0.31
9. Vla	50	M	Irr, 1977	FSH, LH	15	2.75
10. Lel	52	M	Irr, 1979		16	0.48
11. Wie	31	F	TFS, 1977 Irr, 1977	ACTH, TSH LH, FSH	6	0.23
12. May	63	F	None		16	0.14
13. Dijk	68	F	None		24	0.22
14. Kos	56	F	None		45	0.15
15. Jac	37	F	Irr, 1975		23	0.58
16. Wij	74	F	None		48	1.45
17. Age	71	F	Irr, 1954		7	0.32
18. Goe	45	F	Irr, 1979		14	0.59
19. Kor	46	M	None		95	0.92
20. Mas	54	F	Irr, 1976		17	0.28
21. Zie	41	F	Irr, 1965		47	0.25
22. Kip	65	M	Irr, 1977		29	0.27
23. Ste	64	F	Irr, 1976		9	0.60
24. Pal	41	F	Irr, 1978		11	0.21
25. Tan	44	M	Irr, 1980	ACTH, TSH, LH, FSH	28	0.52
26. Lok	41	M	TSS, 1971	ACTH, LH, FSH	59	0.08
27. Wam	43	M	None		36	0.37
28. Ros	48	M	TSS, 1971	ACTH, TSH, LH, FSH	122	0.05
29. Pel	35	M	TFS, 1966 TFS, 1969 Irr, 1969	ACTH, TSH LH, FSH	40	0.05
30. Sch	67	M	Irr, 1972		6	0.25
31. Bri	54	M	TSS, 1963		30	0.11
32. Kui	56	M	Irr, 1971		23	0.16
33. Jan	47	F	TFS, 1967	ACTH, LH, FSH	24	0.37
34. Eek	35	M	Irr, 1976		6	0.13

[1] TSS, transsphenoidal surgery; TFS, transfrontal surgery; Irr, external irradiation.
[2] Mean of 4 determinations.
[3] Mean of 3 determinations.

All investigations were done on separate days following an overnight fast and were kept in the fasting state during the test procedure. Blood samples were taken from an indwelling cannula introduced in an antecubital vein and kept patent by a slow infusion of physiological saline. A basal GH value was obtained by taking the mean of four GH determinations at 08.30 h (fasting), 13.00 h, 17.00 h and 19.00 h (Table 1).

A basal Prl value was obtained by taking the mean of three fasting levels at 08.30 h on separate days (Table 1).

Bromocriptine was given orally at 8.30 h in a dose of 2.5 mg. Blood samples were taken at -15, 0, 120, 240, 360 and 480 min to separate bromocriptine responders and non-responders as described by others (Belforte et al. 1977; Roelfsema et al. 1979).

According to this test, 17 subjects (nos 1-17) were considered as bromocriptine responders (GH fall ⩽ 50% of baseline value); the 17 remaining subjects as bromocriptine non-responders.

Pimozide was given orally in a dose of 4 mg at 08.30 h. In all patients blood samples were taken at -15, 0, 30, 60, 90, 120 and 150 min as was done in the study by Carmina et al. (1979).

Six bromocriptine responders and 6 bromocriptine non-responders were reinvestigated at least 6 weeks after withdrawal of chronic bromocriptine treatment. At that time plasma GH levels were measured hourly in all patients and plasma Prl levels were measured hourly in 3 bromocriptine responders and 3 bromocriptine non-responders for a period of 11 h after administration of 4 mg pimozide. For this last part of the study 3 male and 3 female normal volunteers aged 22-32 years, served as controls. GH (1 μg/l = 2 mU/l) was measured by radioimmunoassay using the SORIN kit (Sorin Biomedica, Saluggia, Italy) with a standard calibrated on the first IRP-HGH (MRC 66/217).

The lower limit of sensitivity was approximately 1 mU/l; intra- and inter-assay variations were 6 and 7.9% (n = 31) respectively.

Prl was measured by radioimmunoassay (commercial IRE-kit). The intra- and inter-assay variations were 7 and 11%, respectively. The values are expressed as U/l (25 ng/ml = 1 IU/l MRC 71/222). Normal basal levels in our laboratory are < 0.6 U/l in females and < 0.55 U/l in males.

RESULTS

The mean basal GH level in the 34 patients with active acromegaly ranged from 6-122 mU/l (Table 1). The mean basal Prl level ranged from 0.05-2.75 U/l (Table 1). Basal Prl was elevated in 6 of 17 bromocriptine responders (35%) and in 2 of 17 bromocriptine non-responders (12%). After the administration of 2.5 mg bromocriptine GH levels were reduced by an average of 67% (range 50-89%) in 17 bromocriptine responders (Table 2) and by an average of 33% (range 16-46%) in 14 non-responders; in 5 non-responders (no. 24, 28, 32, 33, 34) the GH levels even increased (Table 3). After administration of 4 mg pimozide, plasma GH levels showed an average decrease of 15 % (range 0-55%) and an average increase of 14% (range 0-42%) in the group of 'bromocriptine responders' (Table 2).

In the non-responder group plasma GH levels decreased with an average of 14% (range 0-36%) and increased with an average of 20% (range 0-118%) after the test dose of pimozide (Table 3).

In only 1 patient (no. 2). a decrease of the GH level of more than 50% of the base-line value occurred after the test dose of pimozide. This patient belonged to the responder-group and showed a decrease of 88% of the GH level after the administration of bromocriptine.

After the administration of 4 mg pimozide in 6 bromocriptine responders (no. 1, 4, 8, 9, 13, 16) GH levels, measured hourly during 11 h, showed an average decrease of 23% (range 4-45%) and an average increase of 32% (range 0-58%) whereas the same test in 6 bromocriptine non-responders showed an average decrease of 16% (range 0-36%) and an average increase of 57% (range 0-117%)(Table 4). Thus, similar results were obtained in both test periods of 150 min and 11 h.

The mean Prl levels (± SEM) decreased from 0.77 U/l (± 0.17) to 0.15 U/l (± 0.04) in the 17 bromocriptine responders and from 0.34 U/l (± 0.06) to 0.08 U/l (± 0.02) in the 17 bromocriptine non-responders after administration of 2.5 mg bromocriptine. The mean Prl levels (± SEM) showed no change (0.81 ± 0.22 vs. 0.86 ± 0.23 in the 17 bromocriptine responders and 0.28 ± 0.05 vs. 0.30 ± 0.06 in the 17 bromocriptine non-responders) before and 150 min after administration of 4 mg pimozide. When Prl levels were measured during 11 h, an average rise of 67% (range 28-94%) was found in 3 bromocriptine responders (patient no. 8, 13, 16) and an average rise of 93% (range 12-214%) was found in 3 bromocriptine non-responders (patient no. 18, 20, 24) after administration of 4 mg pimozide (Table 5).

When 4 mg pimozide was given to 6 normal volunteers a strikingly higher average Prl rise of 948% (range 358-2050%) was found during 11 h in comparison with the acromegalic patients (Table 5).

DISCUSSION

A paradoxical inhibitory effect of the dopaminergic system on the release of growth hormone in acromegaly has been well documented (Liuzzi et al. 1974, 1978; Chiodini et al. 1975; Wass et al. 1977).

Schwinn et al. (1977) reported that the anti-dopaminergic drug pimozide counteracted the inhibitory effect of bromocriptine on GH secretion in some acromegalics.

Table 2. **Plasma GH levels in 17 bromocriptine sensitive acromegalic patients after administration of bromocriptine (2.5 mg orally) and pimozide (4 mg orally)**

Patient no.	Drug	GH (mU/L), min										Maximal response (%)
		-15	0	30	60	90	120	150	240	360	480	
1	bromocriptine		27				7		3	4	6	-89
	pimozide		25	20	22	25	21	18				-28
2	bromocriptine	56	49				7		7	6	9	-88
	pimozide	32	29	29	21	13	20	20				-55
3	bromocriptine		120				130		31	23	22	-82
	pimozide		87	75	99	104	96	124				-14, +42
4	bromocriptine	29	29				22		7	6	7	-79
	pimozide	46	44	35	37	41	39	43				-20
5	bromocriptine		54				33		16	13	13	-76
	pimozide		55	52	59	66	69	74				+34
6	bromocriptine	55	58				26		16	15	23	-74
	pimozide	67	74	74	61	69	55	53				-28
7	bromocriptine	8	7				4		2	2	3	-71
	pimozide	7	9	7	8	9	7	8				-22
8	bromocriptine	16	13				6		4	5	6	-69
	pimozide	16	10	11	11	12	13	12				+30
9	bromocriptine	11	12				7		4	4	4	-66
	pimozide	13	12	13	14	14	15	17				+42
10	bromocriptine	20	20				13		20	16	7	-62
	pimozide	14	14	13	17	16	14	17				-07, +21
11	bromocriptine	8	8				7		3	4	5	-62
	pimozide	9	8	7	8	8	7	7				-12
12	bromocriptine	14	13				5		6	7	6	-58
	pimozide	16	15	11	12	13	12	13				-27
13	bromocriptine	25	19				13		8	12	16	-58
	pimozide	29	23	24	27	22	19	19				-17
14	bromocriptine	59	57					36	27	25	42	-56
	pimozide	49	55	52	48	43	51	44				-20
15	bromocriptine	27	22				22		12	15	10	-54
	pimozide	20	14	17	14	18	15	17				+28
16	bromocriptine	28	18				12		10	9	10	-50
	pimozide	59	33	38	45	34	42	41				+36
17	bromocriptine	8	8				5		4	7	6	-50
	pimozide	10	7	7	7	6	7					-14

Table 3. Plasma GH levels in 17 bromocriptine insensitive acromegalic patients after administration of bromocriptine (2.5 mg orally) and pimozide (4 mg orally)

Patient no.	Drug	GH (mU/L), min										Maximal response (%)	
		−15	0	30	60	90	120	150	240	360	480		
18	bromocriptine	12	13				9		7	9	12	−46	
	pimozide	13	12	13	13	12	13	12				−04,	+04
19	bromocriptine	83	78				58		43	45	61	−45	
	pimozide	83	79	85	81	88	98	96					+24
20	bromocriptine	13	11				8		6	6	6	−45	
	pimozide	14	10	15	15	15	17	15					+70
21	bromocriptine	39	34				28		19	27	45	−44	
	pimozide	33	34	33	31	32	29	32				-15	
22	bromocriptine	24	23				18		13	15	17	−43	
	pimozide	41	31	30	32	30	28	25				-19	
23	bromocriptine	7	7				4		6	6	4	−43	
	pimozide	8	5	5	6	5	5	4				-20,	+20
24	bromocriptine		11				9		7	12	9	-36,	+09
	pimozide		11	7	10	12	24	20				-36,	+118
25	bromocriptine		24				19		17	17	22	-29	
	pimozide		23	17	16	19	20	17				-30	
26	bromocriptine	82	66				48		75	50	47	-29	
	pimozide	84	60	60	76	60	53	54				-12,	+27
27	bromocriptine	22	25				20		18	19	25	-28	
	pimozide	25	28	28	23	21	22	25				-25	
28	bromocriptine	159	136				109		105	185	99	-27,	+25
	pimozide	125	123	138	120	112	130	126				−09,	+11
29	bromocriptine	51	39				45		31	29	39	-26	
	pimozide	51	53	55	60	58	61	59					+15
30	bromocriptine	5	5				5		4	4	5	-20	
	pimozide	4	6	4	5	5	5	5				-33	
31	bromocriptine	32	32				30		30	27	29	-16	
	pimozide	39	35	39	44	49	49	44					+40
32	bromocriptine	15	16				16		20	18	20		+25
	pimozide	23	21	20	20	18	21	18				-14	
33	bromocriptine	21	19				27		20	20	20		+24
	pimozide	21	22	20	19	21	22	23				-14,	+07
34	bromocriptine	8	6				7		6	7	9		+50
	pimozide	6	7	7	7	7	6	6				-14	

Table 4. Plasma GH levels in 6 bromocriptine responders and 6 bromocriptine non-responders after administration of pimozide (4 mg orally) during 11 h

Patient no.	0	1	2	3	4	5	6	7	8	9	10	11	Maximal response (%)
	Bromocriptine responders GH (mU/l), h												
1	37	30	38	35	34	31	37	28	39	25	23	30	-38, +05
4	60	54	57	63	65	77	75	83	83	92	95	77	-10, +58
8	17	16	15	14	13	18	15	17	23	18	16	17	-23, +35
9	27	26	27	27	29	31	28	34	38	32	27	31	-04, +40
13	20	20	17	16	13	17	15	11	12	14	13	15	-45,
16	25	30	22	24	34	21	31	30	34	30	26	39	-19, +56
	Bromocriptine non-responders GH (mU/l), h												
18	11	9	9	9	9	10	9	9	9	10	10	9	-18,
20	11	12	13	11	16	17	14	13	13	13	14	14	+54
21	37	41	38	34	45	47	51	46	63	58	55	59	-08, +70
24	6	5	5	5	13	5	4	4	4	4	4	5	-33, +117
26	52	69	61	80	53	33	40	45	41	46	40	44	-36, +54
31	38	37	46	46	53	53	56	54	47	46	39	41	-03, +47

Table 5. Plasma Prl levels in 3 bromocriptine responders and 3 bromocriptine non-responders after administration of pimozide (4 mg orally) during 11 h

Patient no.	0	1	2	3	4	5	6	7	8	9	10	11	Maximal response (%)
					Bromocriptine responders (Prl U/l), h								
8	0.24	0.24	0.23	0.28	0.39	0.43	0.40	0.37	0.37	0.33	0.29	0.28	+79%
13	0.17	0.15	0.19	0.24	0.33	0.28	0.32	0.30	0.26	0.26	0.24	0.24	+94%
16	1.83	1.82	1.70	1.88	2.10	2.05	2.11	2.18	2.01	2.04	2.09	2.34	+28%
					Bromocriptine non-responders (Prl U/l), h								
20	0.47	0.46	0.54	0.57	0.85	1.13	1.46	1.20	1.47	1.34	1.20	1.00	+213%
18	0.86	0.77	0.81	0.86	0.91	0.97	0.94	0.96	0.97	0.87	0.86	0.87	+12%
24	0.40	0.36	0.32	0.36	0.43	0.51	0.62	0.56	0.56	0.53	0.48	0.45	+55%

Plasma Prl levels in 3 male and 3 female normal volunteers after administration of pimozide (4 mg orally) during 11 h

Controls	0	1	2	3	4	5	6	7	8	9	10	11	Maximal response (%)
M 1	0.17	0.27	0.29	0.48	0.78	0.77	0.70	0.68	0.42	0.41	0.41	0.37	+358%
M 2	0.11	0.15	0.12	0.32	0.51	0.71	0.55	0.47	0.52	0.37	0.31	0.24	+545%
M 3	0.29	0.37	0.61	0.56	1.20	1.30	1.20	0.85	0.74	0.65	0.62	0.63	+348%
F 4	0.29	0.41	0.38	0.85	2.00	2.70	2.50	1.90	2.10	1.50	1.00	1.10	+831%
F 5	0.26	0.35	0.73	1.50	1.50	3.00	4.00	4.30	2.30	3.10	2.00	1.80	+1554%
F 6	0.20	0.18	0.39	1.90	3.20	4.30	3.30	2.40	2.20	1.50	1.20	1.00	+2050%

Paracchi et al. (1977) found a decrease of plasma GH after acute administration of the antidopaminergic drug sulpiride in 5 acromegalics who also showed a suppression of plasma GH by acute administration of L-dopa and bromocriptine. Schaison et al. (1974) found a decrease of plasma GH during a glucose tolerance test in 5 out of a group of 9 acromegalic patients on chronic sulpiride treatment.

More recently Carmina et al. (1979) demonstrated a decrease of plasma GH levels of more than 50% of the base-line value at 120 min after a test dose of 2 mg pimozide in 4 of 5 bromocriptine insensitive acromegalic patients; a similar response was obtained in only 1 of 6 bromocriptine sensitive patients. On the basis of these results the authors proposed that bromocriptine insensitive acromegalics are characterized by an uninterrupted hypothalamic control of GH secretion which may explain the responsiveness to antidopaminergic drugs.

We have measured the plasma GH response to a single dose of 4 mg pimozide in 17 bromocriptine sensitive and 17 bromocriptine insensitive patients with active acromegaly either untreated or inadequately treated by surgery and/or radiotherapy in a similar way as was reported by Carmina et al. (1979). There was no difference in the plasma GH response to pimozide administration in both groups and with one exception in no case a decrease of the plasma GH level to less than 50% of the base-line value was observed. It is likely that the observed changes can be considered as spontaneous fluctuations of the GH level. Thus, we were unable to reproduce the results reported by Carmina et al. (1979). However, resorption of orally administered pimozide is slow and peak plasma levels appear as late as 3-8 h after drug administration (McCreadie et al. 1979; Pinder et al. 1976). We therefore also measured the plasma GH response to a single oral dose of 4 mg pimozide for a prolonged period of 11 h in 6 bromocriptine responders and in 6 bromocriptine non-responders. Again no difference was found between both groups and in no case a decrease of the plasma GH level to less than 50% of the base-line value was obtained.

Prolactin levels tended to be higher in bromocriptine responders than in bromocriptine non-responders as has been reported before (Lamberts et al. 1982). As could be expected Prl levels decreased in all 34 patients after administration of 2.5 mg bromocriptine.

No changes were observed of the Prl levels in 34 patients after administration of pimozide during 150 min, whereas a moderate increase was found in 6 patients when Prl levels were measured during 11 h. However, this response can be considered as blunted in comparison with the response of 6 normal volunteers. This finding is in agreement with two other studies in which the Prl response to two different dopamine-antagonists (metoclopramide, domperidone) was reported blunted in respectively 10 and 17 acromegalic patients (Spitz et al. 1980; Camanni et al. 1982). As explanations for this blunted response can be considered a dysfunction of central dopaminergic tone or reduced Prl reserve.

The present study confirms the presence of an abnormal dopaminergic control of GH and Prl secretion in acromegaly but does not lend support to the idea that there is a fundamental difference in the degree of hypothalamic dopaminergic control of GH secretion or Prl secretion between bromocriptine sensitive and bromocriptine insensitive patients with acromegaly.

REFERENCES

Belforte L, Camanni F, Chiodini PG, Liuzzi A, Massara F, Molinatti GM, Müller EE & Silvestrini F (1977): Long-term treatment with 2 Br-alpha-ergocryptine in acromegaly. Acta Endocrinol (Copenh) 85: 235-248.

Camanni F, Massara F, Santia M, Molinatti GM & Müller EE (1982): Impaired prolactin responsiveness to dopamine antagonists in acromegaly. Metabolism 31: 1090-1095.

Carmina E, Lo Coco R, Lanzara P & Janni A (1979): Effect of the acute administration of haloperidol and pimozide on plasma GH-levels in acromegaly. Acta Endocrinol (Copenh) 91: 609-615.

Chiodini PG, Liuzzi A, Botalla L, Müller EE, Oppizzi G & Silvestrini F (1975): Stable reduction of plasma growth hormone (hGH) levels during chronic administration of 2-Br-alpha-ergocryptine (CB 154) in acromegalic patients. J Clin Endocrinol Metab 40: 705-708.

Ishibashi M & Yamaji T (1978): Effect of thyrotropin-releasing hormone and bromo-ergocryptine on growth hormone and prolactin secretion in perfused pituitary adenoma tissues of acromegaly. J Clin Endocrinol Metab 47: 1251-1256.

Lamberts SWJ, Liuzzi A, Chiodini PG, Verde S, Klijn JGM & Birkenhäger JC (1982): The value of plasma prolactin levels in the prediction of the responsiveness of growth hormone secretion to bromocriptine and TRH in acromegaly. Eur J Clin Invest 12: 151-155.

Liuzzi A, Chiodini PG, Botalla L, Silvestrini F & Müller EE (1974): Growth hormone (GH)-releasing activity of TRH and GH-lowering effect on dopaminergic drugs in acromegaly: homogeneity in the two responses. J Clin Endocrinol Metab 39: 871-876.

Liuzzi A, Chiodini, PG, Oppizzi G, Botalla L, Verde S, De Stefano L, Colussi G, Gräf KJ & Horowski R (1978): Lisuride hydrogen maleate: evidence for a long lasting dopaminergic activity in humans. J Clin Endocrinol Metab 46: 196-202.

McCreadie RG, Heykants JJP, Chalmers A & Anderson AM (1979): Plasma pimozide profiles in chronic schizophrenics. Br J Clin Pharmacol 7: 533-534.

Paracchi A, Ferrari C & Faglia G (1977): Reduced serum growth hormone levels after acute sulpiride administration in some acromegalic patients. Acta Endocrinol (Copenh) Suppl 212: 274 (abstr).

Pelkonen R, Ylikahri R & Karonen SL (1980): Bromocriptine treatment of patients with acromegaly resistant to conventional therapy. Clin Endocrinol (Oxf) 12: 219-224.

Pinder RM, Brogden RN, Sawyer PR, Speight TM, Spencer R & Avery GS (1976): Pimozide: a review of its pharmacological properties and therapeutic uses in psychiatry. Drugs 12: 1-40.

Roelfsema F, Goslings BM, Frölich M, Moolenaar AJ, van Seters AP & van Slooten H (1979): The influence of bromocriptine on serum levels of growth hormone and other pituitary hormones and its metabolic effects in active acromegaly. Clin Endocrinol (Oxf) 11: 235-244.

Sachdev Y, Tunbridge WMG, Weightman DR, Gomez-Pan A, Duns A & Hall R (1975): Bromocriptine therapy in acromegaly. Lancet 2: 1164-1168.

Schaison G, Croisier JC, Nathan C & Dreyfus G (1974): Essai de traitement de l'acromegalie par le sulpiride. Ann Endocrinol (Paris) 35: 103-110.

Schwinn G, Dirks H, McIntosh C & Köbberling J (1977): Metabolic and clinical studies on patients with acromegaly treated with bromocriptine over 22 months. Eur J Clin Invest 7: 101-107.

Spitz IM, Barzilai D, Luboshitzky R (1980): Diminished prolactin reserve in acromegaly. Metabolism 29: 880-884.

Thorner MO, Chait A, Aitken M, Benker G, Bloom SR, Mortimer CH, Sanders P, Stuart Mason A & Besser GM (1975): Bromocriptine treatment of acromegaly. Br Med J 1: 299-303.

Wass JAH, Thorner MO, Morris DV, Rees LH, Stuart Mason A, Jones AE & Besser GM (1977): Long-term treatment of acromegaly with bromocriptine. Br Med J 1: 875-878.

Wass JAH, Clemmons DR, Underwood LE, Barrow I, Besser GM & van Wyk JJ (1982): Changes in circulating somatomedin-C levels in bromocriptine-treated acromegaly. Clin Endocrinol (Oxf) 17: 369-377.

CHAPTER VII

Long-term follow-up of five untreated acromegalic patients

J.W.R. Nortier, R.J.M. Croughs, J.H.H. Thijssen, and F. Schwarz

Department of Endocrinology, University Hospital, State University of Utrecht, 3500 CG Utrecht, The Netherlands

ABSTRACT

The present study describes the clinical, biochemical and radiological follow-up of 5 patients with acromegaly, selected from a group of 53 patients, who did not receive treatment during a follow-up period of 5-16 years. The characteristics of these patients included: 1) older age (4 cases), 2) a long history of mild symptoms and signs (4 cases), 3) absence of diabetes mellitus, anterior pituitary insufficiency and visual field defects (5 cases), 4) relatively low plasma GH levels (3 cases).

The following observations were made during follow-up:

1. Clinical activity remained constant in 3 patients and lessenned in 2 patients;
2. The lateral fossa area as calculated from a plain lateral X-ray of the skull remained constant;
3. Plasma GH levels measured during an oral glucose tolerance test remained constant in 3 cases, decreased substantially in one case and reached low levels in another case. In this last patient a reproducible increase of plasma GH was found after oral administration of a single dose of 2.5 mg bromocriptine, suggesting complete normality of GH secretion.

It is concluded that acromegaly not necessarily progresses in all patients. The results re-emphasize the importance of taking the spontaneous course of pituitary adenomas into account when assessing the effect of various treatment protocols.

INTRODUCTION

The syndrome of acromegaly was first described as a clinical entity by Marie

Acta Endocrinologica 1984, 106 (in press)

(1886). Its clinical features, presentation and complications are well documented. However, the natural history of the disorder is not accurately known. A reduced life expectancy has been reported by Wright et al. (1970) who analyzed the causes of death in 55 of a group of 194 acromegalic patients from five separate hospitals and by Alexander et al. (1980) who analyzed the causes of death in 45 of a group of 164 acromegalics who were detected in a community survey of a population of 3.1 million over a period of 12 years. In both studies overall mortality rates were higher in untreated than in treated patients. Basal GH levels are positively correlated with the size of the pituitary tumour and young acromegalic patients generally have more rapidly growing and larger tumours at the time of diagnosis than older patients (Melmed et al. 1983; Jadresic et al., 1982).

In the present study the spontaneous course of acromegaly is reported in 5 patients who did not receive any treatment during a median follow-up of 8 years (range 5-16 years) after the diagnosis was made on the basis of abnormal GH values after a glucose load. Reasons for withholding treatment in these patients were, firstly, a long history of mild symptoms and signs (4 cases), secondly, absence of diabetes mellitus, anterior pituitary insufficiency and visual field defects (5 cases) and thirdly, relatively low plasma GH levels (3 cases).

PATIENTS AND METHODS

Clinical details of the 5 patients are shown in Table 1. The diagnosis of acromegaly was based on the patient's history and physical examination and confirmed in all cases by typical radiological findings and by inadequate suppression of plasma GH after a glucose load (lowest plasma GH level more than 4 mU/l). The mean plasma GH levels of the measurements at 0, 30 and 90 min during an oral glucose tolerance test (OGTT) at the time of the first biochemical diagnosis and during follow-up are shown in Fig. 1. Glucose tolerance was assessed according to the criteria of the National Diabetes Data Group (1979). During the last year of follow-up a basal prolactin (Prl) was obtained by taking the mean of three fasting levels measured on separate days.

Thyroidal and gonadal status were assessed by measuring thyroxine (T_4), a resin uptake and calculating the free thyroxine index, basal FSH, LH and either testosterone in men or oestradial (E_2) and oestrone (E_1) in women at the time of biochemical diagnosis and at regular intervals thereafter.

During the last year of follow-up, a TRH-test (200 µg iv) was performed in all patients, an LRH-test (100 µg iv) in the 2 male patients and plasma cortisol was measured at 09.00 a.m. in all patients. Symptoms or signs of hypocorticism were absent in all patients at any time during follow-up.

No patient received any drug therapy during the period of follow-up of which effect on the GH secretion could be expected. Visual fields were studied at the time of biochemical diagnosis of acromegaly and at regular intervals thereafter. The lateral fossa area was calculated from a plain lateral X-ray of the skull taken at the time of biochemical diagnosis and during the last year of follow-up. In addition, basal cisternography with air was performed in patients nos. 1, 2 and 5 directly after biochemical diagnosis of acromegaly and computerized tomography (CT) was performed in patients nos. 1, 2 and 4 at the end of follow-up (Philips tomoscan 300).

The response to the oral administration of 2.5 mg bromocriptine was measured in patient no. 5 during the 16th year of follow-up. This test was performed in the fasting state and was repeated after 3 months. Blood samples were taken from an indwelling cannula introduced in an antecubital vein every 2 h during a period of 8 h.

GH (1 μg/l = 2 mU/l MRC 66/217) and Prl (25 ng/ml = 1 IU/l MRC 71/222) were measured as reported before (Nortier et al., 1983). Throughout the period of follow-up the same reagents were used for the GH-assay.

T_4, resin uptake, TSH, cortisol, LH, FSH, E_1, E_2 and testosterone were measured as reported before (Bijlsma et al., 1982, 1983; Thijssen et al., 1980).

RESULTS

When acromegaly was diagnosed biochemically, the 3 female patients (nos 1, 3 and 4) were over the age of 55 years, the 2 male patients (nos 2 and 5) were respectively 49 and 36 years old. In no patient severe symptoms were present when plasma GH levels were measured for the first time; in one patient (no. 4) acral swelling had already regressed spontaneously. In no case diabetes mellitus was present; hypertension was present in 3 patients, but could easily be controlled by medical therapy.

Thyroid functions as determined by the free T_4 index were normal at any time during follow-up in all patients. A normal TSH response to 200 μg TRH was found in patients nos. 1, 2, 4 and 5 during the last year of follow-up, whereas a flat response was seen in patient no. 3. Basal levels of FSH and LH were in the post-menopausal range in patients nos. 1, 3 and 4 with low oestrogen levels during the last year of follow-up; basal levels of testosterone were normal in patients nos. 2 and 5 at any time during follow-up, a normal response of LH and FSH to LRH was found during the last year of follow-up. Morning cortisol levels were normal during the last year of follow-up in all patients. Visual fields were repeatedly normal in all patients. Calculated from a standard lateral radiographic projection of the pituitary fossa an increased lateral area was found in all patient when 130 mm^2 was considered as the upper limit of normal (Jadresic et al., 1982). At the end of follow-up no

Table 1. Clinical data of 5 acromegalic patients

Patient no.	Sex	Age (yrs)	Duration of acromegaly, at time of diagnosis (years)	Duration of follow-up from bio-chemical diagnosis (years)	Hypertension	Glucose tolerance	Basal Prl[1] (U/l)	Pituitary fossa[2]	Prominent symptoms
1. Wij	F	75	23	12	mild	impaired glucose tolerance	2.0	lateral fossa area 234 mm^2 (A) 247 mm^2 (B) floor assymetrically depressed; basal cisternography: no suprasellar extension; CT: hypodens intra-sellar tumor	enlargement of fingers and feet at age of 40; mild hyperhidrosis from the age of 50; mild headache and tiredness from the age of 63; no progression of symptoms since the age of 65
2. Joo	M	57	13	8	-	impaired glucose tolerance	0.16	lateral fossa area 192 mm^2 (A) 195 mm^2 (B) basal cisternography: no suprasellar extension; CT: isodens pituitary gland; no adenoma visible	widening of wedding-ring at age of 36 and 48; mild tiredness and hyper-hidrosis from the age of 52; no progression of symptoms since the age of 53.
3. May	F	63	4	7	mild	normal	0.20	lateral fossa area 140 mm^2 (A) 130 mm^2 (B)	coarsening of the face since the age of 52; widening of wedding-ring at age of 56; moderate hyperhidrosis from the age of 52; no progression of symptoms since the age of 58.

4. Dij	F	68	14	5	moderate	normal	0.21	lateral fossa area 234 mm^2 (A) 238 mm^2 (B) floor asymmetrically depressed; CT: isodens pituitary tumor invading sphenoidal sinus	coarsening of the face and enlargement of fingers at the age of 49, which worsened until the age of 61; thereafter regression of acral swelling; moderate hyperhidrosis and tiredness from the age of 55, which remained constant until the age of 68.
5. Wi	M	52	7	16	–	normal	0.12	lateral fossa area 340 mm^2 (A) 352 mm^2 (B) floor asymmetrically depressed; basal cisternography: no suprasellar externsion	enlargement of mandible at age of 29; widening of wedding-ring at age 34; regression of acral swelling during the last 10 years; no period of severe headache at any time

[1] Mean of 3 determinations measured on separate days during the last year of follow-up.

[2] Measurement of lateral fossa area (length × depth) from a plain lateral X-ray of the skull at the time of biochemical diagnosis (A) and at the end of follow-up (B). Basal cisternography performed shortly after biochemical diagnosis, CT performed during the last year of follow-up (Philips tomoscan 300).

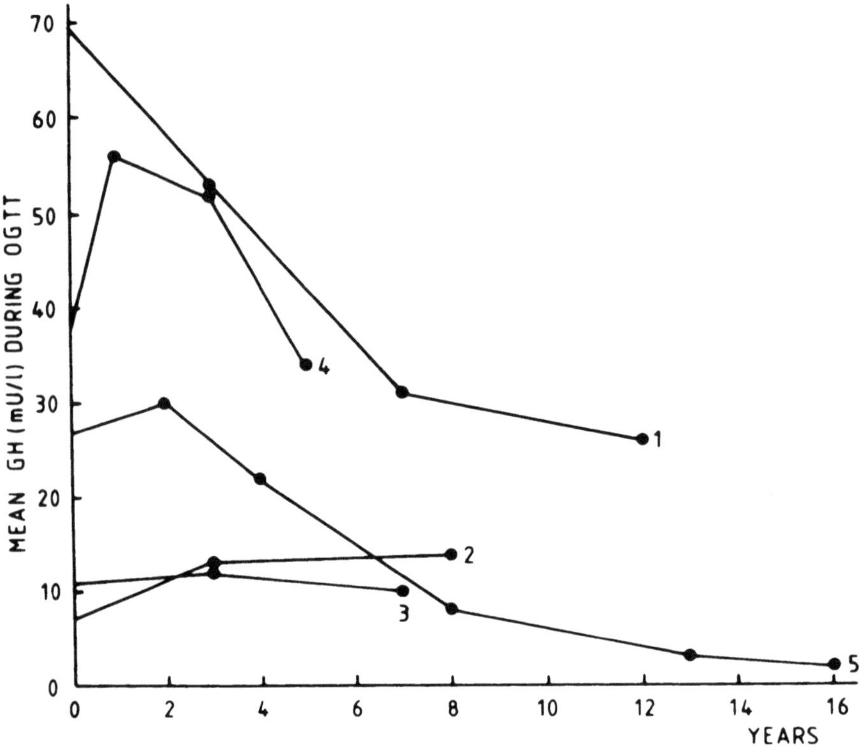

Fig. 1. Mean plasma GH levels during OGTT at 0, 30 and 90 min of 5 acromegalic patients who did not receive any treatment during a follow-up of 5-16 years.

clear differences could be detected in comparison with the period of biochemical diagnosis (Table 1).

In 2 patients (nos. 2 and 3) with slightly elevated plasma GH levels practically no change was observed during follow-up; in one patient (no.4) no change was found of the mean plasma GH level during OGTT at the time of biochemical diagnosis and during the fifth year of follow-up, but during the first and third year of follow-up more elevated levels were found; in 2 patients (nos. 1 and 5) a reduction of the plasma GH levels was observed. Patient no. 5, in whom low plasma GH levels were measured during the 13th year of follow-up, never experienced acute episodes with neurological symptoms or signs suggestive of pituitary apoplexy. During the 16th year of follow-up mean plasma GH levels during OGTT were still low in this patient. A reproducible increase of plasma GH was found at 0, 2, 4, 6 and 8 h after administration of 2.5 mg bromocriptine (respectively 2, 6.5, 13, 5.5, 2 and 2, 8, 14, 6, 3 mU/l).

When only basal plasma GH levels were taken or the mean of the plasma

GH measurements at 30 and 90 min during OGTT similar patterns of the GH secretion could be obtained for all 5 patients as for the mean of GH measurements at 0, 30 and 90 min during OGTT.

DISCUSSION

Acromegaly is a slowly progressive disease and not usually life-threatening (Christy & Warren, 1979) so that use of a drastic therapy does not seem warranted in all patients. However, untreated patients die sooner than they should from the actuarial point of view (Editorial, JAMA 1982, Wright et al., 1970). It is certainly advisable to treat acromegaly early and vigorously in young patients who usually have larger and perhaps more aggressive tumours and in those patients with either high GH values, large tumours or with diabetes mellitus (Jadresic et al., 1980). However, it is well established that circulating GH levels may not correlate with the severity of the disease (Mims & Bethune, 1974; Kanis et al., 1974).

Little is known on the spontaneous course of pituitary adenomas. Recently it was suggested that a substantial proportion (25%) of so-called 'silent' pituitary adenomas undergo spontaneous necrosis without a syndrome of pituitary apoplexy or subsequent pituitary deficiencies (Lindholm et al., 1983). It is generally accepted that microprolactinomas may not progress over years (Nabarro, 1982) and eventually regress or become inactive at older age.

Patients with acromegaly have usually progressed beyond the micro-adenoma stage by the time the condition is diagnosed or treatment is instituted (Laws et al., 1979). The terms 'inactive' or 'burnt out' acromegaly refer to the occasional patient with a spontaneous cure of the clinical picture which has been ascribed to the occurrence of an apoplexy in the pituitary tumour in most cases (Jefferson & Rosenthal, 1959; Weisberg, 1977; Rigolosi et al., 1968). Only in a few studies a subset of acromegalic patients are mentioned who have not received any treatment. Hunter et al. (1974) reported on long-term changes of plasma GH levels in 23 untreated acromegalic patients during periods up to 4 years, but in that study clinical activity and tumour size were not taken into account. Moreover, only 7 patients were followed for more than one year and 4 of these 7 patients for more than 2 years. Variations of plasma GH-levels between -25 and +50% were observed in 10 patients, between -50 and +100% in 8 patients and even greater than that in 5 patients. Williams et al. (1975) reported on the experience in the management of 100 cases of acromegaly; in 17 cases the condition was considered not sufficiently severe to warrant treatment but no follow-up data of these patients are given. Eastman et al. (1979) reported on clinical data of 9 untreated acromegalic patients out of a group of 65; in one patient pituitary apoplexy occurred one week before planned radiotherapy; 4 patients, 2 of whom refused treatment, died 1-5 years after initial work-up; in one patient radiotherapy was pending after hypertension and osteoarthritis had worsened during a follow-up of 12 years; in 3 patients radiotherapy was pending after a short follow-up. From the retrospective studies of Wright et al. (1970) and Alexander et al. (1980) it is not clear how the untreated patients differed from the treated patients with respect to age, tumour mass, plasma GH levels or metabolic consequences of GH hypersecretion.

At our department we analyzed the biochemical and clinical data of 53 patients in whom acromegaly was diagnosed in the period of 1953-1981 and who were still alive in 1982. Of these patients, 23 received conventional external irradiation, 25 underwent pituitary surgery, followed by external irradiation in 11 of these. In 5 patients no treatment was instituted during a follow-up of respectively 5, 7, 8, 12 and 16 years. In no patient a rise of the mean plasma GH during OGTT was observed at the end of follow-up. One patient was of special interest as plasma GH levels decreased to low levels during the 13th year of follow-up; during the 16th year of follow-up a rise of plasma GH was seen after administration of the dopamine agonist bromocriptine. This phenomenon is characteristic of normal regulation of GH as has been demonstrated by Camanni et al. (1975). Presently, the other 4 patients are treated with the dopamine agonist bromocriptine which has resulted in some clinical improvement with a reduction of the mean plasma GH level during the day of more than 50% in 3 of them (nos. 1, 2 and 3).

Although the number of patients in our study is too small to allow any firm conclusion to be drawn about the frequency of spontaneous remission, it appears that acromegaly does not necessarily progress in all patients during a follow-up of 5-16 years. Of course, it cannot be excluded that during longer follow-up plasma GH levels will rise and complications due to GH hypersecretion will occur.

We conclude that in most patients in whom the diagnosis of acromegaly has been made, a therapy must be instituted which is aimed at normalizing GH secretion but that treatment can be withheld in some patients who show either little clinical activity or have rather low plasma GH level, have a limited tumour mass with normal visual fields and are of older age. However, as it is not possible to predict the future course at the time of diagnosis of acromegaly, careful follow-up is necessary when it is decided not to treat the patient.

REFERENCES

Alexander L, Appelton D, Hall R, Ross WM, Wilkinson R (1980): Epidemiology of acromegaly in the Newcastle region. Clin Endocrinol (Oxf) 12: 71-79.

Bijlsma JWJ, Duursma SA, Thijssen JHH & Huber O (1982): Influence of nandrolondeconate on the pituitary-gonadal axis in male. Acta Endocrinol (Copenh) 101: 108-112.

Bijlsma JWJ, Duursma SA, Roelofs JMM & der Kinderen PJ (1983): Thyroid function and bone turnover. Acta Endocrinol (Copenh) 104: 42-49.

Camanni F, Massara F, Belforte L & Molinatti GM (1975): Changes in plasma growth hormone levels in normal and acromegalic subjects following administration of 2-bromo-alpha-ergocriptine. J Clin Endocrinol Metab 40: 363-366.

Christy NP & Warren MP (1979): Disease syndromes of the hypothalamus and anterior pituitary. In: De Groot LJ, Cahill GF Jr, Martini L, Nelson DH, Odell WD, Potts JT Jr, Steinberger E & Winegrad AI (eds). Endocrinology. Grune & Stratton Inc, New York. pp. 215-251.

Eastman RC, Gorden P & Roth J (1979): Conventional supervoltage irradiation is an effective treatment for acromegaly. J Clin Endocrinol Metab 48: 931-940.

Editorial (1982): Choosing the best treatment for acromegaly. JAMA 247: 1320.

Hunter WM, Gillingham FJ, Harris P, Kanis JA, McGurk FM, McLelland J & Strong JA (1974): Serial assays of plasma growth hormone in treated and untreated acromegaly. J Endocrinol 63: 21-34.

Jadresic A, Banks LM, Child DF, Diamont L, Doyle FH, Fraser TR & Joplin GF (1982): The acromegaly syndrome. Q J Med 51: 189-204.

Jefferson M & Rosenthal FD (1959): Spontaneous necrosis in pituitary tumors. Lancet I: 342-344.

Kanis JA, Gillingham FJ, Harris P, Horn DB, Hunter WM, Redpath AT & Strong JA (1974): Clinical and laboratory study of acromegaly: assessment before and one year after treatment. Q J Med 43: 409-431.

Laws ER, Piepgras DG, Randall RV & Abboud CF (1979): Neurosurgical management of acromegaly. J Neurosurg 50: 454-461.

Lindholm J, Bjerre P, Riishede J, Gyldensted C & Hagen C (1983): Pituitary function in patients with evidence of spontaneous disappearance of a pituitary adenoma. Clin Endocrinol (Oxf) 18: 599-603.

Marie P (1886): On two cases of acromegaly: marked hypertrophy of the upper and lower limbs in the head. Revue de Medecin 6: 297-333.

Melmed S, Braunstein D, Horvath E, Ezrin C & Kovacs K (1983): Pathophysiology of acromegaly. Endocr Rev 4: 271-290.

Mims RB & Bethune JE (1974): Acromegaly with normal fasting growth hormone concentrations but abnormal growth hormone regulation. Ann Intern Med 81: 781-784.

Nabarro JDN (1982): Pituitary prolactinomas. Clin Endocrinol (Oxf) 17: 129-155.

National Diabetes Data Group (1979): Classification and diagnosis of diabetes mellitus and other categories of glucose tolerance. Diabetes 28: 1039-1059.

Nortier JWR, Croughs RJM, Donker GH, Thijssen JHH & Schwarz F (1983): No acute effect of pimozide on the plasma GH levels in acromegaly. Acta Endocrinol (Copenh) 103: 461-468.

Rigolosi RS, Schwartz E & Glick SM (1968): Occurrence of growth hormone deficiency in acromegaly as a result of pituitary apoplexia. N Engl J Med 279: 362-364.

Thijssen JHH, van den Berg JHM, Adlercreutz H & Gijzen AHJ (1980): The determination of cortisol in human plasma: evaluation and comparison of seven assays. Clin Chim Acta 100: 39-46.

Weisberg LA (1977): Pituitary apoplexy: association of degenerative change in pituitary adenoma with radiotherapy and detection by cerebral computed tomography. Am J Med 63: 109-115.

Williams RA, Jacobs HS, Kurtz AB, Milar JGB, Oakley NW, Spathis GS, Sulway MJ & Nabarro JDN (1975): The treatment of acromegaly with special reference to trans-sphenoidal hypophysectomy. Q J Med 44: 79-98.

Wright AD, Hill DM, Lowry C & Russell Fraser T (1970): Mortality in acromegaly. Q J Med 34: 1-16.

CHAPTER VIII

General discussion

The aim of the present study was to evaluate the role of medical treatment in the management of acromegaly. On the basis of the results of the studies described in the previous chapters, the questions asked in the introductory chapter will be answered and incorporated in a broader context.

1. *Is the result different if the GH suppressive effect of bromocriptine is evaluated by measurement of plasma GH levels at fixed intervals during the day or if plasma GH is measured during OGTT's and how critical is the time-interval between the last dose of bromocriptine and the performance of an OGTT?*

The evidence of the effectiveness of bromocriptine on the GH secretion in acromegalics is controversial. In some studies a high percentage of successful treatment ranging between 75-90% of the patients has been reported (1-5), while in other reports the results have been rather disappointing with less than 25% responsive acromegalics (6-8). This discrepancy might be due to different methods of evaluation of the GH suppressive effect of bromocriptine (respectively measurement of the plasma GH level at fixed intervals during the day or during an OGTT). The use of an OGTT has been criticized because it does not test physiological control of GH (9). Furthermore bromocriptine has a short duration of action, thus the time-interval between the last dose of bromocriptine and the performance of an OGTT may be critical.

In chapter II the GH suppressive effect of bromocriptine is studied in 12 acromegalics using plasma GH day-profiles as well as OGTT's during continued bromocriptine administration and OGTT's at two different time-intervals after the last dose of bromocriptine. If the OGTT was performed one hour after the last dose, measurement by both methods was equally effective as indicators of the GH suppressive effect of bromocriptine. However, when the OGTT was performed 10 hours after the last dose and a fortiori 34 hours after the last dose misleading results were obtained. The negative results of one major multi-centre placebo controlled study (8) can be explained by a lack of standardization in the time-interval between the last dose of bromocriptine and the performance of an OGTT during chronic bromocriptine therapy.

2. *What is the effect of chronic bromocriptine therapy on the GH secretion and on subjective and objective criteria of clinical activity in patients with still active acromegaly after previous pituitary surgery and/or radiotherapy?*

Part of the controversy about the efficacy of chronic bromocriptine therapy may be due to variations in the daily regimen and dose and to different biochemical and clinical criteria of successful treatment used by various investigators. As the maximal GH suppressive effect of bromocriptine occurs between 4-6 hours and a rebound as early as 10 hours after acute withdrawal has been observed (chapter II), the drug should be prescribed in four divided doses during the day preferably during meals. The daily dose varies from 10-60 mg in the various studies. In one large study of 73 patients (2) a further decrease of the plasma GH levels was found in 12 of 21 patients by increasing the dose from 20-60 mg. However, in another large study of 30 patients good results have been reported with a daily dose of 20 mg (4). In five studies a considerable decrease of the plasma GH level was found with a dose of 20 mg bromocriptine and a further decrease by increasing the dose to 40-60 mg occurred rarely (1,3,10-12). In the study described in chapter III a maximal daily dose of 20 mg bromocriptine was used.

The biochemical and clinical effect of chronic bromocriptine therapy was evaluated in 27 patients with still active acromegaly despite previous treatment with surgery and/or radiotherapy. In accordance with most studies patients who showed a reduction of the mean plasma GH level during the day of more than 50% were arbitrarily defined GH responders. In this way 11 patients could be considered GH responders; in a further 8 patients mean plasma GH levels decreased by more than 25 %.

The clinical response was evaluated by a subjective score of symptoms and by objective criteria of clinical activity such as glucose tolerance, urinary hydroxyproline excretion and finger circumference. In 19 of 27 patients (70%) a good correlation was found between changes of the mean plasma GH level and symptoms. Discordant changes were found in 8 patients, but in 2 of these patients the mean plasma GH level was low and in 2 other patients the score of symptoms was low, which made it difficult to demonstrate any change. Glucose tolerance improved significantly ($p < 0.01$) in 10 GH responders and urinary hydroxyproline excretion decreased significantly ($p < 0.05$) in 8 GH responders. No significant reductions were found in respectively 16 and 14 GH non-responders. Ring size decreased on average 3 mm in the GH responder group and 1.8 mm in the GH non-responder group.

The correlation between GH responsiveness and subjective and objective criteria of clinical activity was better than has been reported in some other studies (2,4,13). Side-effects of bromocriptine were generally mild and included early temporary complaints of nausea and postural hypotension and long-term complaints of constipation and digital vasospasm. In no patient it was necessary to stop treatment because of side-effects.

3. *What is the value of four predictive criteria in combination or separately (i.e. acute bromocriptine test, TRH-test, somatostatin infusion and basal Prl) with respect to the effect of chronic bromocriptine therapy on the GH secretion?*

This question was also discussed in chapter III. A good correlation was present between the GH response to a single dose of 2.5 mg bromocriptine and to chronic bromocriptine therapy ($r = 0.52$, $p < 0.01$). Acute bromocriptine suppression and a TRH test were of equal value in predicting the plasma GH response to chronic bromocriptine therapy (sensitivity respectively 83 and 82%, specificity respectively 69 and 63%). The combination of the TRH test and the bromocriptine test predicted the response to chronic bromocriptine treatment with the same sensitivity but with higher specificity (81%). The data on the predictive value of the bromocriptine test and TRH test are in agreement with other studies (3,4,10). The better information obtained by the combination of the TRH test and bromocriptine test has not been reported before.

Somatostatin infusion gave no additional information as to the chance of success of chronic bromocriptine treatment (sensitivity 73%, specificity 44%).

Hyperprolactinemia was present in 6 patients. Five of these 6 patients belonged to the group of GH responders. Thus, hyperprolactinemia predicted GH responsiveness with high specificity (94%). Responsiveness to TRH and bromocriptine in the acute test was found in all 6 hyperprolactinemic patients. The relation between hyperprolactinemia and responsiveness of acromegalic adenomas to TRH and bromocriptine is controversial. Our data are in accordance with 3 reported studies by Lamberts et al. (14-16), but are in disagreement with 3 other studies (17-19).

Even with the combination of a TRH and bromocriptine test there remains about 20% of normoprolactinemic acromegalic patients who will profit from chronic bromocriptine therapy and who are not recognized by these tests. A short trial of chronic bromocriptine therapy should therefore be given to each patient in whom medical therapy is considered.

4. *Is measurement of somatomedin-C superior to measurement of plasma GH levels in the assessment of the clinical response to chronic bromocriptine therapy in acromegaly?*

In chapter IV the biochemical response to chronic bromocriptine therapy was evaluated in 31 acromegalics by use of the mean of 4 plasma GH determinations during the day and of plasma Sm-C concentrations. The clinical response was evaluated by two methods: 1) a subjective score of symptoms and 2) a combined subjective and objective clinical and metabolic improvement score. Changes in plasma GH levels correlated better with both methods of clinical evaluation than changes in Sm-C values. In some patients clinical improvement was not accompanied by a decrease of plasma GH concentrations but in these Sm-C levels also remained unchanged. These results do not confirm the findings of Wass et al. (5) who suggested that Sm-C concentrations correlate better with clinical status than plasma GH levels. Our data are more in agreement with two other studies (20,21), in which clinical activity correlated better with plasma GH levels than with Sm-C values.

It is difficult to find an explanation for these conflicting results. One of the two methods of clinical evaluation we used was identical to the method used by Wass et al. (5). Also the assay method for Sm-C in our study did not differ essentially from the method used by Wass et al. (5); he only did not use acid chromatography to separate Sm-C from its binding proteins.

Parallel to the Sm-C determinations by Endocrine Sciences, somatomedin A (Sm-A) was measured in 10 patients by a placental radio-receptor assay. Good correlations were found between basal levels before and at the end of the treatment period ($r = 0.71$, $p < 0.01$ and $r = 0.97$, $p < 0.001$) as well as between the change during chonic bromocriptine therapy ($r = 0.74$, $p < 0.01$).

Our investigations lead to the conclusion that measurement of Sm-C is certainly not superior to determination of plasma GH levels in the follow-up of clinical activity in bromocriptine treated acromegaly.

5. *What is the influence of chronic bromocriptine therapy in acromegaly on the different molecular forms of GH? Does the change of the biologically most active monomeric form of GH provide a better correlation than the change of total GH to the clinical response and to the change of somatomedin-C?*

To answer this question Sephadex G 100 chromatography was performed on the plasma of 11 acromegalic patients before and at the end of the treatment period with bromocriptine. The clinical response was evaluated by the same clinical and metabolic improvement score as used in chapter IV. The results of the fractionation studies are described in chapter V. Heterogeneity of plasma GH was confirmed with a major peak of immunoreactivity corresponding to a molecular weight of 20.000 to 22.000 (little GH) and in general two minor peaks corresponding to a MW of 40.000 to 60.000 (big GH) and more than 100.000 (big big GH). Additionally, some immunoreactivity was measured in elution volumes corresponsing to molecular sizes smaller than little GH. It is questionable whether these fractions represent fragments which have retained some immunoreactivity or whether they are artefacts.

Little GH decreased significantly more than big GH. This preferential decrease of little GH in comparison to larger molecular forms is in accordance with one previous study (22) and has been used to explain clinical improvement out of proportion to the reduction in GH secretion (5,22). However, in the 2 patients with clinical improvement without a reduction of GH or Sm-C levels, in whom we carried out fractionation studies, no selective reduction of little GH was found.

The clinical response to bromocriptine therapy in these 11 patients correlated also better with plasma GH levels than with Sm-C values similar to the results obtained in the 31 patients described in chapter IV. The correlation between Sm-C and little GH was not better than that with total GH. It is concluded that measurement of little GH is not superior to determination of total plasma GH in the follow-up of clinical activity in bromocriptine treated acromegaly.

6. *Is there a fundamental difference in the degree of hypothalamic dopaminergic control of GH secretion or Prl secretion between bromocriptine sensitive and bromocriptine insensitive patients with acromegaly?*

It has been suggested in 1979 by Carmina et al. (23) that bromocriptine insensitive acromegalics are characterized by an uninterrupted hypothalamic control of GH secretion and that the GH levels could then be reduced by anti-dopaminergic drugs such as pimozide. He demonstrated that the plasma GH level decreased by more than 50% at 120 minutes after administration of a test dose of pimozide in 4 of 5 bromocriptine insensitive patients, whereas a similar response was obtained in only 1 of 6 bromocriptine sensitive patients. In chapter VI we measured the plasma GH response to a test dose of pimozide in 17 bromocriptine sensitive and in 17 bromocriptine insensitive acromegalics in a similar way. Since the resorption of pimozide after oral administration is slow, we measured plasma GH levels also during a longer period in a smaller group of patients. No difference was found in the GH response to pimozide between bromocriptine responders and non-responders.

As the Prl secretion most closely follows the central dopaminergic tone, the Prl response to pimozide was also measured in bromocriptine responsive and bromocriptine unresponsive acromegalic patients and compared to that in normal subjects. In comparison to the response in normal subjects the Prl response to pimozide was blunted in the acromegalic patients but no difference was observed between bromocriptine sensitive and insensitive patients. These facts suggest an abnormality in the central dopaminergic tone in acromegaly, but there appears to be no difference between bromocriptine responders and non-responders.

7. *Does acromegaly always show clinical, biochemical and radiological progression when treatment is withheld?*

In chapter VII we report on the clinical, biochemical and radiological follow-up of 5 patients with acromegaly, who did not receive treatment during a follow-up period of 5-16 years. At the time of biochemical diagnosis these patients were characterized by older age (4 cases), absence of diabetes mellitus, anterior pituitary insufficiency and visual field defects (all cases) and relatively low plasma GH levels (3 cases). During the follow-up period clinical activity remained constant in 3 patients and decreased in 2. The lateral fossa area as calculated from a plain lateral X-ray of the skull remained constant. Plasma GH levels measured during OGTT remained constant in 3 cases, decreased substantially in 1 case and even reached low levels in 1 case suggestive of normalization of GH secretion. On the basis of the observations in these 5 patients it can be concluded that acromegaly does not necessarily progress in untreated patients and may even show spontaneous decrease of clinical activity.

Although a reduced life expectancy has been reported in acromegaly (24-26) and overall mortality rates are higher in untreated than in treated patients, it is not clear from the reported studies (24,25) how the untreated patients differed from the treated patients with respect to age, tumour mass, plasma GH levels or metabolic consequences of GH hypersecretion. It seems justified in some patients, particularly of older age and with mild clinical activity, to withhold treatment, if close supervision of clinical and biochemical parameters can be maintained.

CONCLUDING REMARKS AND FUTURE PROSPECTS

The dopamine agonist bromocriptine is an effective drug in the treatment of acromegaly but should usually be given as adjunctive therapy next to surgery and/or irradiation since GH secretion is usually not normalized. Only in a few hyperprolactinemic acromegalic patients radiographic evidence of tumour shrinkage has been reported during chronic bromocriptine treatment (27-31). Presumably these were tumours containing both GH and Prl producing cells.

The GH suppressive effect of bromocriptine can be evaluated by GH day profiles or by GH measurements during OGTT if performed during continued bromocriptine administration. The most effective dose of bromocriptine appears to be 20 mg daily divided in 4 doses during the day. Some patients may need up to 60 mg daily to reach the optimal effect. Approximately 70% of patients benefit from chronic bromocriptine therapy with a substantial reduction in GH secretion and in most of them there is clinical improvement as well.

The combination of a bromocriptine test and TRH test has the highest predictive value with respect to the results of chronic bromocriptine therapy. Hyperprolactinemia seems to be associated with GH responsiveness to bromocriptine although this is not generally accepted. The clinical response correlates better with plasma GH levels than with Sm-C concentrations. The biologically most active monomeric form of GH (little GH) is preferably reduced by bromocriptine, but the clinical response does not correlate better with little GH than with total GH. In some patients clinical improvement is noted out of proportion to the GH fall. In our investigations this occurred in 6 cases. In none of them there was a disproportionate reduction of Sm-C. Fractionation of plasma GH was done in 2 of these patients but no decrease of little GH without decrease of total GH was found. There is no evidence that patients who do not respond to bromocriptine will respond to anti-dopaminergic drugs as there is no difference in dopaminergic control of GH or Prl secretion in bromocriptine responders or non-responders.

Recently it was demonstrated that the effects of two other ergot derivatives (lisuride and pergolide) are similar to that of bromocriptine (32-34). Lisuride must also be given in 4 divided doses during the day and its side-effects do not differ from those of bromocriptine. Pergolide is a longer acting dopamine agonist and is effective when given once daily suppressing GH for at least 22 hours (36). The optimal dose is probably 500-1000 mcg daily but further studies are needed to confirm this. No major side-effects have been observed when the drug was slowly step-wise increased. [. . .].

The most rational pharmacological approach in the medical management of acromegaly would be the physiological inhibitor of GH somatostatin. However, the usefulness of somatostatin is limited by its short duration of action. Moreover, it has to be administered parenterally and it causes multiple effects in other systems.

The development of a somatostatin analogue SMS 201-995 (mini-somatostatin) is of interest (37). It has a long-lasting preferential GH suppressive effect in acromegalic patients and causes no rebound after withdrawal (38). The optimal effect is probably obtained by a subcutaneous injection twice daily. This preparation holds promise as another form of adjunctive medical therapy particularly in acromegalic patients who do not respond to dopamine agonists. Further long-term studies are needed to confirm its usefulness.

REFERENCES

1. Sachdev Y, Tunbridge WMG, Weightman DR, Gomez-Pan A, Duns A, Hall R (1975): Bromocriptine treatment in acromegaly. Lancet 2: 1164-1168.
2. Wass JAH, Thorner MO, Morris DV, Rees LH, Stuart-Mason A, Jones AE & Besser GM (1977): Long-term treatment of acromegaly with bromocriptine. Br Med J 1: 875-878.
3. Schwinn G, Dirks H, McIntosh C & Köbberling J (1977): Metabolic and clinical studies on patients with acromegaly treated with bromocriptine over 22 months. Eur J Clin Invest 7: 101-107.
4. Belforte L, Camanni F, Chiodini PG, Liuzzi A, Massara F, Molinatti GM, Müller EE & Silvestrini F (1977): Long-term treatment with 2 Br-alpha-ergocryptine in acromegaly. Acta Endocrinol (Copenh) 85: 235-248.
5. Wass JAH, Clemmons DR, Underwood LE, Barrow I, Besser GM & Van Wyk JJ (1982): Changes in circulating somatomedin-C levels in bromocriptine-treated acromegaly. Clin Endocrinol (Oxf) 17: 369-377.
6. Summers VK, Hipklin LJ, Diver MJ & Davis JC (1975): Treatment of acromegaly with bromocriptine. J Clin Endocrinol Metab 40: 904-906.
7. Dunn PJ, Donald RA & Espineer EA (1977): Bromocriptine suppression of plasma growth hormone in acromegaly. Clin Endocrinol (Oxf) 7: 273-281.
8. Lindholm J, Riishede J, Verstergaard S, Hummer L, Faber O & Hagen C (1981): No effect of bromocriptine in acromegaly: a controlled trial. N Engl J Med 304: 1450-1454.
9. Thorner MO, Besser GM, Wass JAH, Liuzzi A, Hall R, Müller EE & Chiodini PG (1981): Bromocriptine in acromegaly. N Engl J Med 305: 1092-1093.
10. Roelfsema F, Goslings BM, Frölich M, Moolenaar AJ, VanSeters AP & VanSlooten H (1979): The influence of bromocriptine on serum levels of growth hormone and other pituitary hormones and its metabolic effects in active acromegaly. Clin Endocrinol (Oxf) 11: 235-244.
11. Sachdev Y, Gopal K & Garg VK (1981): Bromocriptine therapy in acromegaly. A long-term review of 35 cases. Postgraduate Med J 57: 210-216.
12. Brooks AP, Stephan PJ, Nairn LM, Strong JA (1979): Bromocriptine and acromegaly: therapeutic implications. J Royal Soc Med 72: 562-564.
13. Halse J, Haugen HN, Bohmer T (1977): Bromocriptine treatment in acromegaly: clinical and biochemical effects. Acta Endocrinol (Copenh) 86: 464-472.
14. Lamberts SWJ, Klijn JGM, Kwa GH & Birkenhäger JC (1979): The dynamics of growth hormone and prolactin secretion in acromegalic patients with "mixed" pituitary tumours. Acta Endocrinol (Copenh) 90: 198-210.
15. Lamberts SWJ, Liuzzi A, Chiodini PG, Verde S, Klijn JGM & Birkenhäger JC (1982): The value of plasma prolactin levels in the prediction of the responsiveness of growth hormone secretion to bromocriptine and TRH in acromegaly. Eur J Clin Invest 12: 151-155.
16. Lamberts SWJ, Klijn JGM, van Vroonhoven CGJ, Stefano SZ & Liuzi A (1983): The role of prolactin in the inhibitory action of bromocriptine on growth hormone secretion in acromegaly. Acta Endocrinol (Copenh) 103: 446-450.
17. Moriondo P, Travaglini P, Rondena M, Beck-Peccoz P, Contin Puglisì F, Ambrosi B & Faglia G (1980): Prolactin secretion in acromegaly. In: Pituitary Microadenomas (eds G Faglia, MA Giovanelli & RM MacLeod). Academic Press, London & New York, pp. 247-255.
18. Faglia G. Travaglini P, Beck-Peccoz P, Ambrosi B, Moriondo P, Elli R & Rondena M

(1980): Anterior pituitary hormones other than those hypersecreted in patients with functioning microadenomas. In: Pituitary microadenomas (eds G Faglia, MA Giovanelli & RM MacLeod). Academic Press, London & New York, pp. 277-294.
19. Nieuwenhuijzen Kruseman AC, Bots GThAM, Roelfsema F, Frölich M & van Dulken H (1983): Immunocytochemical growth hormone and prolactin in pituitary adenomas causing acromegaly and their relationship to basal serum hormone levels and the growth hormone response to thyrotrophin releasing hormone. Clin Endocrinol (Oxf) 19: 1-8.
20. Moses AC, Molitch ME, Sawin CT, Jackson IMD, Biller BJ, Furlanetto R, Reichlin S (1981): Bromocriptine therapy in acromegaly: use in patients resistant to conventional therapy and effect on serum levels of somatomedin-C. J Clin Endocrinol Metab 53: 752-758.
21. Stonesifer LD, Jordan RM, Kohler PO (1981): Somatomedin-C in treated acromegaly: Poor correlation with growth hormone and clinical response. J Clin Endocrinol Metab 53: 931-934.
22. Benker G, Sandmann K, Tharandt L, Hackenberg K, Reinwein D (1979): Gel filtration studies of serum growth hormone in acromegaly following bromocriptine administration. Horm Res 11: 151-160.
23. Carmina E, Lo Coco R, Lanzara P & Janni A (1979): Effect of the acute administration of haloperidol and pimozide on plasma GH-levels in acromegaly. Acta Endocrinol (Copenh) 91: 609-615.
24. Wright AD, Hill DM, Lowy C & Russell Fraser T (1970): Mortality in acromegaly. Q J Med 34: 1-16.
25. Alexander L, Appleton D, Hall R, Ross WM & Wilkinson R (1980): Epidemiology of acromegaly in the Newcastle region. Clin Endocrinol (Oxf) 12: 71-79.
26. Editorial (1982): Choosing the best treatment for acromegaly. JAMA 247: 1320.
27. Wass JAH, Thorner MO, Charlesworth M, Moult PJA, Dacie JE, Jones AE (1979): Reduction of pituitary-tumor size in patients with prolactinomas and acromegaly treated with bromocriptine with and without radiotherapy. Lancet ii: 66-69.
28. Corenblum B, Hanley DA (1981): Bromocriptine reduction of prolactinoma size. Fertility & Sterility 36: 716-719.
29. Spark RF, Baker R, Bienfang DC, Bergland R (1982): Bromocriptine reduces pituitary tumor size and hypersecretion. "Requiem for pituitary surgery?" JAMA 247: 311-316.
30. Prescott RWG, Kendall-Taylor P, Hall K, Johnston DG, Crombie A & McGregor A (1982): Hyperprolactinemia in men – response to bromocriptine therapy. Lancet i: 245-248.
31. McGregor AM, Scanlon MF, Hall R, Hall K (1979): Effects of bromocriptine on pituitary tumour size. Br Med J 3: 700-703.
32. Liuzzi A, Chiodini PG, Oppizzi G, Botalla L, Verde S, De Stefano L, Colussi G, Gräf KJ & Horowski R (1978): Lisuride hydrogen maleate: evidence for a long-lasting dopaminergic activity in humans. J Clin Endocrinol Metab 46: 196-202.
33. Verde S, Chiodini PG, Liuzzi A (1980): Effectiveness of the dopamine agonist lisuride in the treatment of acromegaly and pathological hyperprolactinemic states. J Endocrinol Invest 4: 405-414.
34. Marek J, Sramkova J, Schullerova M, Stephan J & Schreiberova O (1981): Long-term treatment of acromegaly with lisuride: differences of effect on growth hormone and somatomedin. Endokrinologie 78: 175-185.
35. Kleinberg DL, Boyd AE, Wardlaw S (1983): Pergolide for the treatment of pituitary tumors secreting prolactin or growth hormone. N Engl J Med 309: 704-709.
36. Kendall-Taylor P, Upstill-Goddard G, Cook D (1983): Long-term pergolide treatment of acromegaly. Clin Endocrinol (Oxf) 19: 711-719.
37. Bauer W, Briner U, Doepfner W, Haller R, Huguenin R, Marback P, Petcher TJ & Pless J (1982): SMS 205-995: A very potent and selective octapeptide analogue of somatostatin with prolonged action. Life Sciences 31: 1133-1140.

38. Plewe G, Neufeld M, Krause U, Oppermann D, Beyer J (1984): Suppression of GH-secretion to normal values by a long-acting analogue of somatostatin in acromegaly. Acta Endocrinol (Copenh) 105, suppl 264: 30.

Summary

In 1886 Pierre Marie described two patients who had a striking non-congenital hypertrophy of the extremities. He named the condition "acromegaly" from the Greek akron (= extremity) and megas (= great). It was later discovered that the disorder was caused by hypersecretion of growth hormone (GH) from the pituitary gland. After a short outline of the historical background, epidemiology and pathogenesis of acromegaly, the various therapeutic modalities are discussed in chapter I. Transsphenoidal pituitary surgery is the most effective form of treatment. External irradiation is indicated if patients are not cured by surgery. It can also be considered as a primary form of treatment in older patients and in poor surgical risks, but it may last many years before its optimal effect on the GH secretion is reached. Therefore since 1974 the possibility of adjunctive medical therapy with the dopamine agonist bromocriptine has received much attention. However, the reported results with this treatment vary.

The aim of the clinical and biochemical studies described in this thesis was to evaluate the role of adjunctive medical therapy – next to surgery and radiotherapy – in acromegalic patients.

In chapter II two methods of evaluation of the GH suppressive effect of bromocriptine are compared. Measurement of the mean plasma GH level during the day or during OGTT were equally effective indicators of the suppressive effect of bromocriptine treatment on GH secretion in acromegaly if the OGTT was performed one hour after the last dose of bromocriptine. Misleading results were obtained if the OGTT was performed ten hours after the last dose and a fortiori 34 hours after the last dose.

In chapter III the effect of chronic bromocriptine therapy is evaluated. Twenty-seven acromegalic patients with disease still active despite previous treatment with surgery and/or radiotherapy were treated with 10-20 mg bromocriptine for 6-9 months. Mean plasma GH levels decreased by more than 50% in 11 patients (GH responders) and by more than 25% in a further 8 patients. Glucose tolerance decreased significantly ($p < 0.01$) in 10 GH responders and urinary hydroxyproline excretion decreased significantly ($p < 0.05$) in 8 GH responders, whereas no significant decrease was found in respectively 16 and 14 GH non-responders. In 19 of 27 patients (70%) a good correlation was found between changes of the mean plasma GH levels and the change of symptoms.

The GH response to a single dose of 2.5 mg bromocriptine (more than 50% decrease) and the GH response to TRH (more than 100% rise) were of equal value in predicting the plasma GH response to chronic bromocriptine therapy (sensitivity respectively 73 and 82%, specificity respectively (69 and 63%). The combination of these two tests predicted the response to chronic bromocriptine therapy with the same sensitivity but with higher specificity (81%). The degree of GH suppression during somatostatin infusion gave no additional information as to the chance of success of chronic bromocriptine therapy. Hyperprolactinemia predicted the plasma GH response to chronic bromocriptine therapy with high specificity (94%) but with low sensitivity.

In chapter IV the value of the somatomedin-C (Sm-C) determination is assessed in the follow-up of bromocriptine treated acromegalic patients. The biochemical response to chronic bromocriptine therapy in 31 acromegalic patients was evaluated by the mean of 4 plasma GH determinations during the day and by Sm-C concentrations. The clinical response was assessed by two methods: only subjective criteria and a combination of subjective and objective criteria of disease activity. Both methods of clinical evaluation showed a good correlation with each other. Changes in plasma GH levels correlated better with the clinical response than changes in Sm-C. In some patients clinical improvement was recorded without a change in plasma GH levels, but also Sm-C remained unchanged. From this study it was concluded that Sm-C is not superior to GH in following disease activity.

In chapter V changes of the various molecular forms of GH were studied in relation to the clinical response and changes of Sm-C levels by performing Sephadex G-100 gel filtration studies on the plasma of 11 acromegalic patients before and at the end of chronic bromocriptine therapy. It was confirmed that bromocriptine causes a preferential reduction of the biologically most active monomeric form of GH (little GH). However, in the two patients from this group, in whom clinical improvement was noted without a reduction of GH or Sm-C, no selective reduction of little GH was found which could have explained the discrepancy in the clinical and biochemical response. The correlation between the change of little GH with the clinical response and the change of Sm-C was not better than that of total GH.

It has been suggested that bromocriptine insensitive acromegalics are characterized by an uninterrupted hypothalamic dopaminergic control of GH secretion and that the GH levels could then be reduced by antidopaminergic drugs such as pimozide. In the study described in chapter VI the GH response to the administration of a test dose of pimozide was measured in 17 bromocriptine sensitive and 17 bromocriptine insensitive acromegalics. In six patients the Prl response was measured as well and compared with the Prl response to pimozide in normal subjects. There was no difference in the GH and the Prl response to pimozide between bromocriptine sensitive and bromocriptine insensitive patients. In comparison to normal subjects the Prl response to pimozide was blunted in all acromegalic patients suggestive of a dysfunction of dopaminergic regulation or a reduced Prl reserve.

In chapter VII the clinical, biochemical and radiological follow-up is described of five acromegalic patients who were left untreated during a period of 5-16 years because of either mild clinical activity, relatively low plasma GH levels or older age. In no patient biochemical or clinical progression could be documented during this period. These observations re-emphasize the importance of taking the spontaneous course of pituitary adenomas into account when assessing the effect of various treatment modalities.

In the general discussion (chapter VIII) the questions raised in the introductory chapter are answered on the basis of the studies described in the chapters II-VII and incorporated in a broader context. Additionally, some comments are made on future developments of adjunctive medical therapy of acromegalic patients.

Bei Fragen zur Produktsicherheit wenden Sie sich bitte an:
If you have any questions regarding product safety,
please contact:

Walter de Gruyter GmbH
Genthiner Straße 13
10785 Berlin
productsafety@degruyterbrill.com